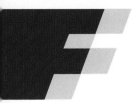

FAST FACTS

Infection Highlights 1997

Indispensable
Guides to
Clinical
Practice

Edited by

Mark H Wilcox

Senior Lecturer in Microbiology and
Consultant Medical Microbiologist,
University of Leeds, Leeds, UK

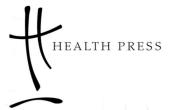

HEALTH PRESS

Oxford

Fast Facts – Infection Highlights 1997
First published 1998

© 1998 Health Press Limited
Elizabeth House, Queen Street, Abingdon,
Oxford, UK OX14 3JR
Tel: +44 (0)1235 523233
Fax: +44 (0)1235 523238

Fast Facts is a trademark of Health Press Limited

A CIP catalogue record for this title is available
from the British Library.

ISBN 1-899541-02-0

Library of Congress
Cataloguing-in-Publication Data

Wilcox, MH. (Mark)
Fast Facts – Infection Highlights 1997/
Mark H Wilcox

Designed and typeset by Hinton Chaundy
Design Partnership, Thame, UK

Printed by Nuffield Press, Abingdon, UK

Introduction

Infection is an expanding specialty that critically impacts on most areas of medicine and surgery. As the number of publications continues to increase, it is inevitable that ever busier clinicians and specialists alike cannot review all the important new data in their fields. One solution to this problem is the provision of abstracted material, but this does not provide the all important overview of a subject. Furthermore, this approach relies on publications having been indexed and catalogued. At the other extreme, review articles are often unwieldy and out of date by the time of publication.

Not only does *Fast Facts – Infection Highlights 1997* provide up-to-date information on a range of key topics within the field, but it places these advances into context, and so allows the reader to decide on their immediate relevance to current practice. The topics covered reflect the far-reaching effects of infection, and chapter authors are renowned experts on their subjects, with access to the latest information such as that only recently released at international meetings.

I hope you enjoy this first *Infection Highlights*, and find it both informative and stimulating. Look out for *Infection Highlights 1998*!

Mark H Wilcox
Editor

Chlamydia trachomatis infection

C Carder and GL Ridgway

Department of Clinical Microbiology, University College London Hospitals, London, UK

Chlamydia trachomatis (Figure 1) is the most common curable bacterial sexually transmitted pathogen in the UK. Over 31,000 new episodes of genital chlamydial infection were reported in Genitourinary Medicine clinics in England and Wales in 1996, with females showing a higher rate than males (Figure 2).[1] In low prevalence populations, up to 50% of men[2] and 70% of women[3] carrying *C. trachomatis* may be asymptomatic. Sequelae of chlamydial genital infection include pelvic inflammatory disease, infertility, ectopic pregnancy, proctitis and reactive arthritis. However, there is generally a lack of knowledge of chlamydial infection amongst people at risk, and current initiatives are aimed at education and ways of determining prevalence in the UK.

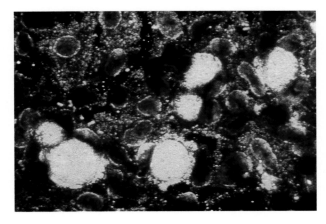

Figure 1

Mature inclusion of *Chlamydia trachomatis* in McCoy cells (Giemsa stained – dark-field examination).

Which method of testing?

The role of nucleic acid amplification technology in the routine diagnosis of *C. trachomatis* infections is evolving rapidly. Two commercial assays are now available for routine use:

- polymerase chain reaction (PCR; Roche Amplicor)
- ligase chain reaction (LCR; Abbott LCx).

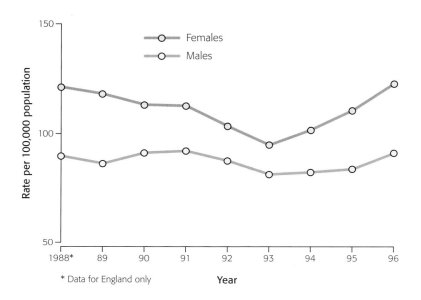

Figure 2 New cases of infection with *Chlamydia trachomatis* seen in genitourinary clinics, 1988–1996.

These techniques have increased sensitivity compared with more traditional tests, such as cell culture and enzyme-linked immunoassays (EIA). Results for both of these amplified DNA techniques have shown a sensitivity and specificity of > 95% and 99%, respectively.[4] In comparison, cell culture has a sensitivity of 65–100% and specificity of 100%. The traditional method of cell culture is in decline, with few laboratories in the UK now offering this service. Even under ideal conditions, cell culture requires meticulous sampling and optimal transport to the laboratory, irrespective of which culture method is to be used.

Commercial PCR and LCR techniques are based on the amplification of plasmid DNA specific for *C. trachomatis* and involve three major steps:

- sample preparation
- DNA amplification
- amplicon detection.

In order to reduce the risk of DNA contamination, the sample preparation area must be separated from the amplification and detection stages. The amplification stage – incorporating separation, annealing, primer extension

Highlights in **Chlamydia trachomatis** infection 1997

WHAT'S IN ?

- Molecular diagnostics
- Urine and vaginal swabs for screening
- Single-dose macrolide therapy – azithromycin
- Quinolone treatment – ofloxacin

WHAT'S OUT ?

- EIA technology
- Routine cell culture

WHAT'S COMING (SOON) ?

- Newer quinolones (shorter course)

WHAT'S COMING (LATER) ?

- Selected-population screening programme

(for PCR) and ligation (for LCR) – takes place in a thermal cycler over 30–40 cycles.

An alternative nucleic acid amplification method, transcription-mediated amplification (TMA; Gen-Probe) is now emerging. TMA is based on the amplification of C. *trachomatis*-specific ribosomal RNA (rRNA). The sensitivity and specificity reported are 91.4% and 99.6% respectively.[5] One advantage of TMA over PCR or LCR is its isothermic amplification stage. This means that a thermal cycler is not used, so separate areas are not needed to prevent cross-contamination of amplicons. There are about 10 copies of the plasmid DNA – the target sequence for PCR and LCR – in each organism, compared with many thousands of copies of rRNA, the TMA target. This initial boost in target sequence availability should, theoretically, enhance the sensitivity of TMA. With the advent of molecular diagnostic technology, it is now appreciated that no single test provides 100% sensitivity and specificity. Currently, nucleic acid amplification methods are proving to be the best tests on the market. There is no need for complacency, however, as further work is required to eliminate test problems, such as inhibitor contamination,[6] reproducibility[7] and hormonal factors,[8] that have played a part in lowering sensitivity.

Concurrent infections are common in patients with sexually transmitted diseases. Some 25% of men and 30–50% of women with *Neisseria gonorrhoeae* are also infected with *C. trachomatis*. A multiplex PCR assay allowing detection of both pathogens is available, with no reported loss in sensitivity or specificity.[9] This would eliminate the need to take multiple samples in the clinic, which would save time and money for both the clinic and the laboratory.

Which site to sample?

Amplified DNA technologies have demonstrated excellent sensitivity and specificity in diagnosing *C. trachomatis* from first catch urine (FCU) samples,[10,11] a specimen from women that was previously considered too insensitive to use. This finding has led to the re-evaluation of the best sampling sites for genital chlamydial infections. The use of patient-obtained vaginal swabs showed a sensitivity of 93.9% compared with 89.9% for cervical swab specimens.[12] Vulval swabs have also been investigated and show a sensitivity of 88.5% compared with 92.3% for FCU.[13]

Which treatment?

The azalide macrolide, azithromycin, is effective against lower genital chlamydial infection as a single 1 g oral dose. As a consequence, compliance is excellent and side-effects are much lower than with erythromycin.[14]

The fluoroquinolone, ciprofloxacin, has proved disappointing for the treatment of genital chlamydial infections. However, ofloxacin is effective at either 300 mg twice daily or 400 mg once daily, given orally for 7 days.[14]

Newer agents, such as the fluoronaphthyridone, trovafloxacin, are also showing encouraging preliminary results. The findings of larger clinical trials, particularly those using shorter treatment courses, are awaited.

There has been a recent resurge of interest in the use of vaginal microbicides with broad-spectrum antiviral and antibacterial activity. One *in-vitro* study with C31G (a mixture of an alkyl betaine and an alkyl dimethyl amine oxide), demonstrated anti-chlamydial activity,[15] although further work remains to be done.

Regardless of the antimicrobial agent chosen, the treatment of partners is a key component in the control of genital chlamydial infections.

Are we ready to screen?

With the increasing use of amplified DNA technology, the higher sensitivities associated with these methods, and the exciting discovery that non-invasive samples are showing impressive results, the time is now ripe to reconsider selected population screening. Genç and Mårdh investigated the cost effectiveness of identifying and treating 1000 asymptomatic female carriers of *C. trachomatis*.[16] They compared screening with no screening and the effects of antimicrobial regimens on the outcome of the screening strategies. They concluded that nucleic acid amplification (NAA) tests combined with single-dose azithromycin treatment of patients found to be positive was the most cost-effective strategy when the prevalence of infection was 6% or more. With a prevalence of less than 6%, there was a trade-off between cost and benefits. Screening with either NAA or EIA added cost, but improved the quality of health care. NAA testing resulted in greater cost per capita, but led to significantly better cure rates than EIA. Compared with no intervention, cell culture was cost effective only when the prevalence of infection was greater than 14%.

Paavonen and colleagues have developed a computer-based model for a more 'thorough' cost-benefit analysis of screening versus no screening, based on PCR testing of FCU specimens in women.[17] They concluded that when the sensitivity of the screening test was 90%, the threshold value for the prevalence of *C. trachomatis* infection was as low as 3.2%. The cost saving increased with increasing prevalence. In a recent study in a low-risk population of women with a prevalence of 2.6%, 74% of the positive women would have been 'captured' if a selective screening programme had tested only those women aged under 25 years with two or more sexual partners in the past year.[18] This would have reduced the total number of women screened from 865 to 295 (35%).

There is still a long way to go before deciding whether a national or selective screening programme will be introduced in the UK. A successful programme has been initiated in Sweden, with a marked reduction in the prevalence of chlamydial infections. The UK Department of Health is currently addressing the inconsistencies of screening, diagnosis and treatment on a national basis.

References

1. Sexually transmitted diseases quarterly report: genital *Chlamydia trachomatis* infection in England and Wales. *Commun Dis Rep CDR Wkly* 1997;7:394–5.

2. Zelin JM, Robinson AJ, Ridgway GL, Allanson-Jones E, Williams P. Chlamydial urethritis in heterosexual men attending a genitourinary medicine clinic: prevalence, symptoms, condom usage and partner change. *Int J STD & AIDS* 1995;6:27–30.

3. Bauwens JE, Clark AM, Leoffelholz MJ, Herman SA, Stamm WE. Diagnosis of *Chlamydia trachomatis* urethritis in men by polymerase chain reaction assay of first catch urine. *J Clin Microbiol* 1993;31:3013–16.

4. Robinson AJ, Ridgway GL. Modern diagnosis and management of genital *Chlamydia trachomatis* infections. *Br J Hosp Med* 1996;55:388–93.

5. Pasternack R, Vuorinen P, Miettinen A. Evaluation of the Gen-Probe *Chlamydia trachomatis* Transcription Mediated Amplification assay with urine specimens from women. *J Clin Microbiol* 1997;35:676–8.

6. Clad A, Naudascher I, Flecken U, Freidank HM, Petersen EE. Evidence of labile inhibitors in the detection of *Chlamydia trachomatis* in cervical specimens by polymerase chain reaction. *Eur J Clin Microbiol Infect Dis* 1996;115:744–7.

7. Peterson EM, Darrow V, Blanding J, Aarnaes S, Maza LM. Reproducibility problems with the Amplicor PCR *Chlamydia trachomatis* Test. *J Clin Microbiol* 1997:135:957–9.

8. Crowley T, Horner P, Hughes A, Berry J, Paul I, Caul O. Hormonal factors and the laboratory detection of *Chlamydia trachomatis* in women, implications for screening. *Int J STD & AIDS* 1997;8:25–31.

9. Mahony JB, Luinstra KE, Tyndall M, Sellors JW, Krepel J, Chernesky M. Multiplex PCR for detection of *Chlamydia trachomatis* and *Neisseria gonorrhoeae* in genitourinary specimens. *J Clin Microbiol* 1995;33:3049–53.

10. Chernesky M, Chong S, Jang D, Luinstra K, Sellors J, Mahony JB. Ability of commercial Ligase Chain Reaction and PCR assays to diagnose *Chlamydia trachomatis* infections in men by testing first void urine. *J Clin Microbiol* 1997;35:982–4.

11. Pasternack R, Vuorinen P, Pitkäjärvi T, Koskela M, Miettinen A. Comparison of manual Amplicor PCR, Cobas Amplicor PCR, and LCx assays for detection of *Chlamydia trachomatis* infection in women by using urine specimens. *J Clin Microbiol* 1997; 35:402–5.

12. Hook E, Smith K, Mullen C *et al.* Diagnosis of genitourinary *Chlamydia trachomatis* infections by using the Ligase Chain Reaction on patient-obtained vaginal swabs. *J Clin Microbiol* 1997;35:2133–5.

13. Stary A, Najam B, Lee H. Vulval swabs as alternative specimens for Ligase Chain Reaction detection of genital chlamydial infection in women. *J Clin Microbiol* 1997;35:836–8.

14. Ridgway GL. Treatment of chlamydial genital infection. *J Antimicrob Chemother* 1997; 40:311–14.

15. Wyrick PB, Knight ST, Gerbig DG *et al.* The microbicidal agent C31G inhibits *Chlamydia trachomatis* infectivity in vitro. *Antimicrob Ag Chemother* 1997;41:1335–44.

16. Genç M, Mårdh PA. A cost-effectiveness analysis of screening and treatment for *Chlamydia trachomatis* infection in asymptomatic women. *Ann Intern Med* 1996;124:1–7.

17. Paavonen J. Is screening for *Chlamydia trachomatis* infection cost effective? *Genitourin Med* 1997; 73:103–4.

18. Grun L, Tassano-Smith J, Carder C *et al.* Comparison of two methods of screening for genital chlamydial infection in women attending in general practice: cross sectional survey. *BMJ* 1997; 315:226–30.

Helicobacter pylori infection

P Moayyedi

Gastroenterology Department, Centre for Digestive Diseases, Leeds General Infirmary and Leeds University, UK

Helicobacter pylori is a Gram-negative organism that has colonized the human stomach for millions of years. It is responsible for more deaths in developed countries than any other infectious disease[1] and yet, until recently, has managed to avoid the prying eyes of microbiologists, histopathologists and clinicians. *H. pylori* was finally thrust into the limelight after it was cultured in 1982, since when it has revolutionized our understanding of gastroduodenal disease.

Epidemiology and transmission
H. pylori is mainly acquired in childhood, particularly in circumstances of socio-economic deprivation and overcrowding. After a brief vomiting illness the infection becomes asymptomatic and chronic, although in some children the organism is spontaneously cleared.[2] The mode of transmission is unclear. The organism can be isolated from faeces and saliva, but there is no consistent epidemiological evidence that *H. pylori* is transmitted by either the faecal–oral or the oral–oral route. The organism can survive in gastric juice,[3] and vomit has been proposed as a vehicle of transmission[4] although studies in this area are lacking.

Diagnosis
Diagnosis of *H. pylori* has traditionally relied on histopathology, microbiology and rapid urease test, all of which require endoscopy and gastric biopsy. Research is now focusing on non-invasive tests, such as the ^{13}C-urea breath tests (^{13}C-UBT), serology and near-patient tests for *H. pylori*. The ^{13}C-UBT is regarded as the most accurate non-invasive test and this has been further enhanced by the introduction of a citric acid test meal.[5] The patient is required to fast for a ^{13}C-UBT, which is inconvenient and considered unnecessary in a recent report.[6] ^{13}CO$_2$ in the breath is detected using a mass spectrometer. This is expensive and cheaper methods

Highlights in **Helicobacter pylori infection** *1997*

WHAT'S IN ?

- Non-invasive tests for *H. pylori*
- Proton pump inhibitor triple therapies
- Screen and treat strategies for young dyspeptics

WHAT'S STILL CONTROVERSIAL ?

- *H. pylori* and extra-gastrointestinal diseases
- Screening and treating *H. pylori* in healthy populations

WHAT'S OUT ?

- Proton pump inhibitor dual therapies
- Treating peptic ulcer disease with anti-secretory drugs

have been developed.[7] Serology is cheap and convenient, but is less accurate than ^{13}C-UBT. Preliminary reports on the accuracy of second generation commercial serology kits, however, are promising.[8] Near-patient *H. pylori* kits can give a diagnosis within 10 minutes and are extremely useful in primary care and out-patient settings. These kits are accurate in some populations,[9] but have poor specificity in others,[10] indicating that local validation is necessary before they are used in clinical practice.

Complications of *H. pylori* infection

H. pylori is the commonest chronic bacterial infection worldwide and remains asymptomatic throughout life in most individuals. The organism is the major cause of duodenal and gastric ulcer, however, and treatment of the infection will cure these diseases. *H. pylori* is also strongly associated with

15

gastric, low-grade B-cell lymphomas; treatment of the infection causes regression of these lesions. Although gastric lymphoma is a rare disease, this interesting finding is evidence that treating an infectious disease may cure a lymphoproliferative disorder. Several case-control studies have demonstrated that *H. pylori* is an important risk factor for gastric neoplasia, the second commonest cause of cancer deaths worldwide. A recent study indicated that in patients with endoscopically treated early gastric cancer, eradication of the infection reduced the risk of developing further neoplasia.[11] This study was not a randomized controlled trial and these are urgently needed to establish whether treatment of *H. pylori* will reduce the risk of developing this important disease. *H. pylori* causes chronic gastritis in all infected individuals and it is possible that long-term, low-grade inflammation may lead to diseases outside the gastrointestinal tract. Indeed, *H. pylori* has been associated with an increased risk of ischaemic heart disease,[12,13] although reports are conflicting.[14] *H. pylori* has also been linked with diminished adult height, psoriasis, urticaria, migraine and acute stroke.[15] This list will undoubtedly keep growing, although most, if not all, of these associations will be found to be spurious.

Pathogenic strains of *H. pylori*

As with most other bacteria, different strains of *H. pylori* have different pathogenicity. Some strains produce a cytotoxin that is closely related to the CagA (cytotoxin associated gene A) protein. Antibodies to CagA are therefore a marker for cytotoxin-producing *H. pylori*. These strains cause more gastric mucosal inflammation and atrophy, duodenal ulcer, gastric ulcer and gastric cancer than CagA-negative infections.[16] Another marker of pathogenicity is the production of a vacuolating cytotoxin encoded by the *VacA* gene. Interestingly, all strains of *H. pylori* possess the *VacA* gene, but only some produce the vacuolating cytotoxin. The reason for this is the variability in the signal sequence and mid-region of the gene. There are two types of signal sequence, *s1* (which is further divided into *s1a* and *s1b*) and *s2*, and two types of mid-region, *m1* and *m2*. *VacA s1/m1* strains produce the highest levels of vacuolating cytotoxin and are most closely associated with peptic ulceration, while *VacA s1/m2* strains produce intermediate levels of cytotoxin. *VacA s2/m2* strains do not produce cytotoxin and are associated with a low risk of peptic ulceration; *VacA s2/m1* strains have not been described.[17] Other potential markers of virulence, such as the *iceA* gene (*i*nduced by *c*ontact with *e*pithelium),[18] have been less well characterized, but may provide insights into the mechanisms by which *H. pylori* causes peptic ulcer disease. CagA production and the *VacA s1/m1* genotype indicate more virulent *H. pylori*, but strains not possessing these markers may still have ulcerogenic and carcinogenic potential. These factors are therefore academically interesting, but are not as yet clinically useful.

Is *H. pylori* infection ever beneficial?

H. pylori has been our companion for millions of years and it is possible that this infection may actually have benefited our ancestors. Infection with *H. pylori* usually results in increased gastric acid secretion, which may have provided additional protection from enteric pathogens.[19] In developed countries with good hygiene standards, this theoretical advantage of *H. pylori* infection is no longer important, but is there any other benefit from having this organism? A study in duodenal ulcer patients treated for *H. pylori* infection suggested that patients in whom therapy was successful were more likely to develop oesophagitis compared with patients having unsuccessful therapy or placebo.[20] The two groups, however, were not comparable, as 58% of the *H. pylori*-positive controls developed peptic ulcer disease during follow-up and were withdrawn from the study, compared with only 2% of *H. pylori*-negative cases.

H. pylori may enhance the protective effect of proton pump inhibitors against non-steroidal anti-inflammatory drug (NSAID)-induced peptic ulceration.[21] A preliminary study suggested that oesophageal adenocarcinoma was less common in patients harbouring CagA strains of *H. pylori*.[22] These observations require further study and at present it is fair to say that the risks of having *H. pylori* far outweigh the benefits.

Therapy for *H. pylori*

Bismuth salts combined with two antibiotics or proton pump inhibitors combined with either amoxycillin or clarithromycin have largely been abandoned as results have been disappointing. Attention has focused on proton pump inhibitors combined with two antibiotics, as these regimens produce eradication rates consistently above 80%. The front runners appear to be a proton pump inhibitor (e.g. omeprazole, 20 mg, or lansoprazole,

30 mg) combined with either clarithromycin, 250 mg bd, and metronidazole, 400 mg bd, (OCM) or clarithromycin, 500 mg bd, and amoxycillin, 1 g bd, (OAC) for 7 days;[23] these regimens usually achieve eradication rates of around 90%. OCM is the most cost-effective treatment in most developed countries, but in areas with a high prevalence of metronidazole-resistant *H. pylori* (>50%), the efficacy of OCM is reduced and OAC becomes the preferred option.[24] Decreasing the length of treatment to 3 or 5 days reduces the efficacy of both regimens.[25,26]

Immunization against *H. pylori* would be the ideal approach to preventing peptic ulcer disease and gastric cancer. Oral immunization is effective in animal models and, interestingly, can also successfully treat animals already infected with the organism.[27] The adjuvants used in these experiments are too toxic for human consumption and oral immunization with recombinant urease without adjuvants has been ineffective in humans.[28] Multiple *H. pylori* antigens combined with a non-toxic adjuvant, such as a modified heat-labile enterotoxin of *Escherichia coli*, are likely to be successful in the future, but the timescale of these developments is uncertain.[29]

H. pylori – who to treat

All patients with a gastric or duodenal ulcer should receive treatment against *H. pylori* if it is present. *H. pylori* eradication is the treatment of choice for low-grade, B-cell gastric lymphoma and may be warranted in patients with a strong family history of gastric cancer.

The European *Helicobacter pylori* Study Group have suggested that a screen and treat strategy may be appropriate for dyspeptic patients under 45 years of age, without sinister symptoms and not taking NSAIDs.[30] Gastric cancer is rare in this age group and *H. pylori*-negative patients are unlikely to have peptic ulcer disease. Those who are *H. pylori* positive may have peptic ulcer disease, but this can be treated by eradication therapy. Preliminary evidence indicates this strategy reduces endoscopy workload whilst detecting significant pathology,[31] although this needs further evaluation.

It is estimated that *H. pylori* causes 1 in 30 deaths in men and 1 in 60 deaths in women, so it is tempting to speculate that screening and treating entire populations may reduce this mortality.[1] Such a policy could be cost effective,[32] but trials are needed to establish that eradication of *H. pylori* reduces the risk of gastric cancer before these strategies can be implemented.

Conclusion

Like all great discoveries, *H. pylori* has created as many questions as it has answered. Scientists have now got *H. pylori* firmly fixed in their sights and hopefully many of the questions posed in this review will be answered by the time this organism is next reviewed in *Infection Highlights*.

References

1. Axon ATR, Forman D. *Helicobacter gastroduodenitis: a serious infectious disease. BMJ* 1997;314:1430–1.

2. Tindberg Y, Blennow M, Granström M. Clinical findings in a cohort of children monitored with *H. pylori* serology from 0.5–11 years of age (abstract). *Gut* 1997;41:A66.

3. Galal G, Wharburton V, West A *et al.* Isolation of *H. pylori* from gastric juice. *Gut* 1997;41:A40.

4. Axon ATR. Review article: Is *Helicobacter pylori* transmitted by the gastro-oral route? *Aliment Pharmacol Ther* 1995;9:585–8.

5. Dominguez-Munoz JE, Leodolter A, Sauerbruch T, Malfertheiner P. A citric acid solution is the optimal test drink in the ^{13}C-urea breath test for the diagnosis of *Helicobacter pylori* infection. *Gut* 1997;40:459–62.

6. Moayyedi P, Braunholtz D, Heminbrough E *et al.* Do patients need to fast for a ^{13}C-urea breath test? *Eur J Gastroenterol Hepatol* 1997;9:275–7.

7. Murnick DE, Peer BJ. Laser-based analysis of carbon isotope ratios. *Science* 1994;263:945–7.

8. Wilcox MH, Dent THS, Hunter JO *et al.* Accuracy of serology for the diagnosis of *Helicobacter pylori* infection. *J Clin Path* 1996;49:373–6.

9. Moayyedi P, Carter AM, Catto A, Heppell RM, Grant PJ, Axon ATR. Validation of a rapid whole blood test for diagnosing *Helicobacter pylori* infection. *BMJ* 1997;314:119.

10. Stone MA, Mayberry JF, Wicks ACB *et al.* Near patient testing for *Helicobacter pylori*: a detailed evaluation of the Cortecs Helisal Rapid Blood test. *Eur J Gastroenterol Hepatol* 1997;9: 257–60.

11. Uemura N, Mukai T, Okamoto S *et al. Helicobacter pylori* eradication inhibits the growth of intestinal type of gastric cancer in initial stage. *Gastroenterology* 1996;110:A282.

12. Patel P, Mendall MA, Carrington D et al. Association of Helicobacter pylori and Chlamydia pneumoniae infections with coronary heart disease and cardiovascular risk factors. BMJ 1995; 31:711–14.

13. Ossei-Gerning N, Moayyedi P, Smith S et al. Helicobacter pylori infection is related to atheroma in patients undergoing coronary angiography. Cardiovasc Res 1997;35:120–4.

14. Rathbone B, Martin D, Stephens J, Thompson JR, Samani NJ. Helicobacter pylori seropositivity in subjects with acute myocardial infarction. Heart 1996;76:308–11.

15. Gasbarrini A, Franceschi F, Gasbarrini G, Pola P. Extraintestinal pathology associated with Helicobacter infection. Eur J Gastroenterol Hepatol 1997;9:23–8.

16. Parsonnet J, Friedman GD, Orentreich N, Vogelman H. Risk for gastric cancer in people with CagA-positive or CagA-negative Helicobacter pylori infection. Gut 1997;40:297–301.

17. Atherton JC, Peek RM, Tham KT, Cover TL, Blaser MJ. Clinical and pathological importance of heterogeneity in vacA, the vacuolating cytotoxin gene of Helicobacter pylori. Gastroenterology 1997;112:92–9.

18. Peek RM, Thompson SA, Atherton JC, Blaser MJ, Miller GG. Expression of iceA, a novel ulcer-associated H. pylori gene, is induced by contact with gastric epithelial cells and is associated with enhanced mucosal IL-8. Gut 1996; 39:A71.

19. Blaser MJ. Not all Helicobacter pylori strains are created and equal: should all be eliminated? Lancet 1997;349:1020–2.

20. Labenz J, Blum AL, Bayerdorffer E, Meining A, Stolte M, Borsch G. Curing Helicobacter pylori infection in patients with duodenal ulcer may provoke reflux esophagitis. Gastroenterology 1997; 112:1442–7.

21. Hawkey CJ, Swannell AJ, Eriksson S et al. Lower frequency of gastroduodenal ulcers and erosions and dyspeptic symptoms in NSAID users during maintenance with omeprazole compared with ranitidine. Gut 1996;39:A69.

22. Chow WH, Blaser MJ, Blot WJ et al. H. pylori and CagA status in relation to risk of adenocarcinomas of oesophagus and stomach by anatomical subsite. Gut 1997;41:A33.

23. Lind T, Veldhuyzen van Zanten S, Unge P et al. Eradication of Helicobacter pylori using one-week triple therapies combining omeprazole with two antimicrobials: The MAC 1 study. Helicobacter 1996;1:138–44.

24. Megraud F, Lehn N, Lind R et al. The MACH-2 Study: Helicobacter pylori resistance to antimicrobial agents and its influence on clinical outcome. Gastroenterology 1997;112:A216.

25. Peitz U, Nusch A, Tillenburg B et al. Impact of treatment duration and metronidazole resistance on H. pylori (HP) cure with omeprazole, metronidazole and clarithromycin. Gastroenterology 1997;112:A255.

26. Moayyedi P, Langworthy H, Tompkins DS, Mapstone N, Chalmers DM, Axon ATR. The optimum 5-day therapy against *Helicobacter pylori*. *Gut* 1997;40:A5.

27. Cuenca R, Blanchard TG, Czinn SJ *et al*. Therapeutic immunization against *Helicobacter mustelae* in naturally infected ferrets. *Gastroenterology* 1996;110:1770–5.

28. Kreiss C, Buclin T, Cosma M *et al*. Oral immunization with recombinant urease without adjuvant in *H. pylori*-infected humans. *Gut* 1997;39:A39.

29. Lee A. Therapeutic immunization against *Helicobacter* infection. *Gastroenterology* 1996;110:2003–6.

30. The European *Helicobacter pylori* Study Group. Current European concepts in the management of *Helicobacter pylori* infection: The Maastricht Consensus Report. *Gut* 1997;41:8–13.

31. Moayyedi P, Clough M, Hemingborough E, Chalmers DM, Axon ATR. Open access ^{13}C-urea breath tests (OA ^{13}C-UBT): comparisons with and impact on open access endoscopy. *Gut* 1996;38:A34.

32. Parsonnet J, Harris RA, Hack HM, Owens DK. Modelling cost-effectiveness of *Helicobacter pylori* screening to prevent gastric cancer: a mandate for clinical trials. *Lancet* 1996;348:150–4.

Escherichia coli O157

MA Neill

Division of Infectious Diseases, Brown University School of Medicine and Memorial
Hospital of Rhode Island, Rhode Island, USA

Since its initial discovery 15 years ago, *Escherichia coli* O157:H7 has
attained the stature of a formidable pathogen. Unlike opportunistic
pathogens, *E. coli* O157:H7 can infect normal healthy individuals of all
ages, though it remains most common in young children. Its short
incubation period (3–5 days) has produced steep epidemic curves in point
source outbreaks. *E. coli* O157:H7 has proven adept at finding novel food
vehicles and in demonstrating the weak links in the current food safety
chain.

Epidemiology

Fresh produce. Several new vehicles for the transmission of *E. coli* O157:H7
have been recognized. Unpasteurized fresh apple juice, distributed across
western USA and Canada, proved to be the vehicle of transmission in an
outbreak among young children.[1] *E. coli* O157:H7 with the same DNA
fingerprint was isolated from unopened containers of Odwalla apple juice,
thus confirming an association with fresh pressed apple cider that had been
suspected in previous outbreaks. This micro-organism may survive for more
than 2 weeks at refrigeration temperatures, even in a highly acidic
environment (pH < 4.6).

Contaminated lettuce has also been implicated as a vehicle for
transmission of *E. coli* O157:H7 infection.[2] Investigation was, however,
unable to determine the point at which the contamination was introduced
(i.e. during processing, on the farm, or at the retail level). A startling recent
discovery has been the link between *E. coli* O157:H7 infection and the
consumption of fresh alfalfa sprouts, a foodstuff commonly regarded as a
health food.[3] Case clusters in widely separated areas in the USA were linked
by molecular subtyping of isolates. This identified a sufficient number of
cases for epidemiological analysis, and a case control study implicated alfalfa
sprouts produced from seeds from the same source. Whether the seeds were

Highlights in **<u>Escherichia coli</u> O157** *in 1997*

WHAT'S IN ?

- New vehicles of transmission
  - fresh produce
  - unpasteurized apple juice ·
- Intestinal carriage by animals other than cattle
- Relatedness of sporadic cases – 'many mini-outbreaks'

WHAT'S IN (STILL) ?

- Fluid/rehydration
- Supportive care

WHAT'S IN AND CONTROVERSIAL ?

- Pasteurization of fresh juices
- Irradiation of fresh produce
- Antibiotic treatment

WHAT'S OUT ?

- Hamburger as main vehicle for transmission
- Sole bovine reservoir
- Bovine vaccination strategy
- Treatment with toxin-binding resin
- Treatment with antimotility agents

contaminated after sprouting or were intrinsically contaminated, as has been previously demonstrated for Salmonella, is unknown.

Regulatory systems must now address these findings and develop preventive strategies. In the case of fresh juices, pasteurization or equivalent technologies are capable of making such products safe. However, for fresh or minimally processed produce, pathogen elimination or reduction is more difficult and this has prompted a new look at the use of irradiation for produce.

Food preparation. A massive outbreak in Japan highlighted the vulnerability of large-scale food preparation and distribution networks. More than 5000 individuals, mainly schoolchildren, were infected with *E. coli* O157:H7. Available evidence suggested that infection was acquired by consumption of contaminated white radish sprouts served as part of a school-lunch programme.[4,5]

Another large scale outbreak that occurred in central Scotland, UK, involved nearly 500 people.[6] Although cooked meat products from a single retail butcher shop were implicated in transmission, epidemiological investigation found that many individuals did not reheat or further cook the food after purchase. People also kept foods for far longer than would have been expected. A major area of concern identified in the Pennington report was the lack of physically separate areas for cooked and raw products, and the lack of complete records enabling the source of foods to be traced back from the retail trade to the wholesale level.[7] The UK Government is examining the findings closely.[8]

Molecular subtyping has played an increasingly prominent role in confirming suspected outbreaks. A seminal study has shown the value of molecular subtyping to identify outbreaks where none was suspected.[9] Molecular subtyping of *E. coli* O157:H7 isolates obtained as part of ongoing surveillance in Minnesota, USA, revealed that many small case clusters ('mini-outbreaks') could be demonstrated when sporadic, apparently unrelated, cases were re-analysed by molecular subtyping. Somewhat disconcertingly, numerous subtypes were observed, suggesting that infections came from multiple sources. These data underscore the need to pursue a primary preventive strategy for *E. coli* O157:H7 in the efforts to control the disease.

Ecology

Previously, *E. coli* O157:H7 had often been associated with outbreaks caused by undercooked hamburgers and, for several years, had been repeatedly isolated from dairy and beef cattle. These findings had largely focused attention on cattle as the major reservoir for this pathogen. More recently,

E. coli O157:H7 has been isolated from several other animal species.[10] Sheep, deer and dogs have all been shown to have naturally occurring faecal excretion of *E. coli* O157:H7, and the bacterium has also been isolated from a horse.[11]

These findings indicate that the natural ecology of *E. coli* O157:H7 is far more complicated than originally envisaged, making it highly unlikely that a vaccination strategy for cattle will be an effective way to remove this pathogen from the food chain.

Treatment

Haemorrhagic colitis caused by *E. coli* O157:H7 infection prompts most patients to seek medical attention. The severity of the illness and the high rate of complications, such as haemolytic uraemic syndrome (HUS), have compelled physicians to seek suitable treatments. An often overlooked intervention is that of adequate hydration, which is not an easy prospect in ill patients with vomiting and diarrhoea. One investigator with considerable clinical experience in this area has, however, stressed the importance of maintaining adequate hydration as a cornerstone of therapy.[12]

At a recent international meeting, the results of a long-awaited trial with the verotoxin-binding resin, Synsorb-Pk, were presented.[13] Synsorb-Pk was administered to patients with bloody diarrhoea while awaiting analysis of stool samples.[14] Disappointingly, administration of Synsorb-Pk had no beneficial effect in either the amelioration of symptoms or in the prevention of HUS.

Several studies have now confirmed that antimotility agents are unhelpful, and are probably harmful, in the treatment of diarrhoea caused by *E. coli* O157:H7.[15,16] Administration of antiperistaltic agents increases the risk of HUS in children with diarrhoea due to *E. coli* O157:H7 and increases CNS involvement in children who develop HUS.

Considerable attention has been focused on the role of antibiotics in the treatment of diarrhoea associated with *E. coli* O157:H7. Antimicrobial agents have been shown to increase the level of detectable toxin, though the magnitude of the effect varies with the chemical class of agent. Some, but not all, retrospective analyses of outbreaks and small case series have shown a detrimental effect of antibiotics. In a retrospective analysis of cases from the 1996 Japan outbreak, antibiotic administration within the first 3 days of illness was associated with a lower overall risk for the development of HUS.[17] In contrast, an analysis of cases from the large outbreak in Washington State, USA, showed no beneficial effect of antibiotic treatment in the first 3 days of illness.[18] The data from Japan are tantalizing, as these are the first data from a large case series suggesting a beneficial role for antibiotics.

It therefore remains to be determined whether antibiotic administration can be demonstrated to have a protective effect in a prospective trial. Currently, a firm conclusion cannot be drawn either to support or refute the use of antibiotics in *E. coli* O157:H7 infection.

References

1. Centers for Disease Control. Outbreak of *Escherichia coli* O157:H7 infections associated with drinking unpasteurized commercial apple juice – British Columbia, California, Colorado and Washington, October 1996. *MMWR* 1996;45(44):975.

2. Ackers M, Mahon E, Leahy T *et al*. An outbreak of *Escherichia coli* O157:H7 infection associated with leaf lettuce consumption, Western Montana. 36th Interscience Conference on Antimicrobial Agents and Chemotherapy, September 15–18, 1997: Abstract K43.

3. Centers for Disease Control. Outbreaks of *Escherichia coli* O157:H7 associated with eating alfalfa sprouts – Michigan and Virginia, June–July 1997. *MMWR* 1997;46(32):741–4.

4. WHO. Prevention and control of enterohaemorrhagic *Escherichia coli* O157:H7 infections. Geneva: WHO, 1997: Document 97.6.

5. Izumiya H, Terajima J, Wada A *et al*. Molecular typing of enterohaemorrhagic *E. coli* O157:H7 isolates in Japan by using pulsed-field gel electrophoresis. *J Clin Microbiol* 1997;35:1675–80.

6. WHO. Prevention and control of enterohaemorrhagic *Escherichia coli* O157:H7 infections. Geneva: WHO, 1997: Document 97.6:13–15.

7. The Pennington Group. Report on the circumstances leading to the 1996 outbreak of infection with enterohaemorrhagic *E. coli* O157:H7 in Central Scotland, the implications for food safety and the lessons to be learned. Edinburgh: HMSO, 1997.

8. Government response to the Pennington report. London: HMSO, 1997.

9. Bender JB, Hedberg CW, Besser JM, Boxrud DJ, MacDonald KL, Osterholm MT. Surveillance for *Escherichia coli* O157:H7 infections in Minnesota by molecular subtyping. *N Engl J Med* 1997;337:388–94.

10. Armstrong GL, Hollingsworth J, Morris JG. Emerging foodborne pathogens: *Escherichia coli* O157:H7 as a model of entry of a new pathogen into the food supply of the developed world. *Epidemiol Rev* 1996;18:29–51.

11. Chalmers RM, Salmon RL, Willshaw GA *et al*. Vero-cytotoxin-producing *Escherichia coli* O157:H7 in a farmer handling horses. *Lancet* 1997;349:1816.

12. Tarr PI. *E. coli* O157:H7: clinical, diagnostic and epidemiological aspects of human infection. *Clin Infect Dis* 1995; 20:1–10.

13. Armstrong GD, Rowe PC. Clinical trials of Synsorb Pk in preventing HUS. Third International Symposium on Shiga-toxin-producing enterohaemorrhagic *Escherichia coli* infections, Baltimore MD, June 22–26, 1997.

14. Armstrong GD, Rowe PC, Goodyer P *et al*. A phase I study of chemically synthesized verotoxin (Shiga-like toxin) Pk trisaccharide receptors attached to Chromosorb for preventing hemolytic uremic syndrome. *J Infect Dis* 1995;171:1042–5.

15. Cimolai N, Carter JE, Morrison BJ, Anderson JD. Risk factors for the progression of *Escherichia coli* O157:H7 enteritis to hemolytic uremic syndrome. *J Pediatr* 1990;116:589–92.

16. Cimolai N, Morrison BJ, Carter JE. Risk factors for the central nervous system manifestations of gastroenteritis associated hemolytic uremic syndrome. *Pediatr* 1992;90:616–21.

17. Takeda T, Tanimura M, Yoshino K *et al*. Questionnaire-based clinical aspects of VTEC infection in Japan, 1996. Third International Symposium on Shiga-toxin-producing *Escherichia coli* infections, Baltimore MD, June 22–26, 1997: Abstract 19.

18. Bell B, Griffin PM, Lozano P *et al*. Predictors of hemolytic uremic syndrome in children during a large outbreak of *Escherichia coli* O157:H7 infections. *Pediatr* 1997;100:127.

Clostridium difficile infection in practice

MH Wilcox

Department of Microbiology, University of Leeds and The General Infirmary, Leeds, UK

Clostridium difficile infection is invariably associated with exposure to antibiotics. As the spores of the bacterium are endemic in many hospital environments, most cases of infection are seen nosocomially. Recent spiralling incidence figures have heightened awareness of this pathogen and highlighted the importance of both traditional infection-control measures and restriction of antibiotic prescribing. For example, in the 4 months following removal of several antibiotics from restricted prescribing status in one US hospital, the *C. difficile* diarrhoea rate almost doubled.[1]

Epidemiology

The most recent figures from the Communicable Disease Surveillance Centre indicate that the incidence of *C. difficile* is continuing to rise; in England and Wales, the total number of reports in the first three-quarters of 1997 was approximately 37% higher than in the same period in 1996.[2] Two recent UK studies have highlighted the burden to healthcare resources posed by *C. difficile* infection.[3,4] Both found marked increases in length of stay (averages of 21 and 17 days), and additional costs attributable to *C. difficile* infection exceeded £4000 per episode.[3] Furthermore, in one of these studies, *C. difficile* infection was found to be significantly associated with mortality in elderly hospitalized patients.[3]

Starr and colleagues have proposed a population model to explain the clinical correlation between antibiotic use and *C. difficile* infection (Figure 1).[5] They argue that four states exist, depending on the combination of susceptibility to infection and colonization status, that can precede symptomatic *C. difficile* infection. The pressures exerted by antibiotic use and environmental exposure may force hospitalized patients towards the symptomatic group. Pressure provided by 'high-risk' antibiotics may be particularly responsible, both in the selection of individuals within a ward setting who have increased susceptibility to *C. difficile* and by increasing the environmental load of bacterial spores (secondary to diarrhoeal

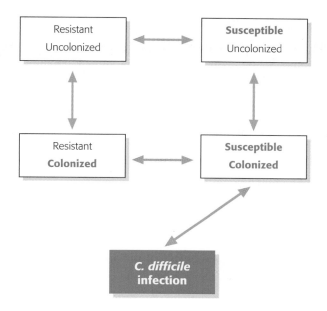

Figure 1 Population model proposed by Starr *et al.*[5] to explain the clinical correlation between antibiotic use and *C. difficile* infection.

contamination). The most successful control strategies for *C. difficile* are likely, therefore, to include both restriction of antibiotic use and procedures to minimize cross-colonization/infection within the ward setting.

Diagnosis

A 4-year study from Switzerland confirmed earlier reports of the marked financial savings that can be realized by only culturing faecal specimens for enteric bacterial pathogens (other than *C. difficile*) from patients hospitalized for up to 3 days.[6] Exceptions included follow-up samples, specimens from immunocompromised patients or those patients initially culture-negative, and rarely in the setting of an institutional food-borne outbreak of infection. For patients on or with a recent history of antibiotic therapy, *C. difficile* toxin testing was the optimal single diagnostic test.

A significantly higher recurrence rate of *C. difficile* infection in HIV-positive patients (26%) compared with non-HIV cases (14%) has recently been reported in Spain.[7] Of particular note, metronidazole resistance was significantly more common in HIV-positive cases (38% versus 15%, respectively). This is the first account of apparent widespread metronidazole resistance in C. *difficile* and confirmation of these findings is important given the problems of antimicrobial susceptibility testing of anaerobes.

Treatment

A recent study compared the efficacies of oral fusidic acid, metronidazole, teicoplanin and vancomycin for the treatment of diarrhoea associated with C. *difficile*.[8] Patient numbers were relatively small (28–31 per group) and the results for the 55–71% of patients in each treatment group who had colitis proven by colonoscopy showed no significant differences between the treatment groups. It was concluded that metronidazole remains the first-line treatment of choice.

New therapeutic options are required and one possibility could be the use of an anti-C. *difficile* bovine immunoglobulin concentrate of colostrum. Following oral administration of this immunoglobulin preparation, human faeces have recently been reported to contain neutralizing antitoxin activity, and results of further human studies are awaited with interest.[9,10] In another approach, two patients non-responsive to metronidazole and vancomycin were successfully treated with pooled intravenous normal human immunoglobulin.[11] Not surprisingly, in view of the high prevalence of anti-C. *difficile* antibodies in healthy adults,[12] the pooled immunoglobulin preparations examined all contained cytotoxin-neutralizing antibodies.[11] Interesting results have also been reported recently from a murine C. *difficile* model, in which high faecal concentrations of bacterial metabolic products were associated with resistance to colonization following an oral challenge of spores.[13] Furthermore, bacterial metabolic products could be increased by raising dietary levels of fermentable fibre.

While it is not uncommon to see patients with multiple symptomatic recurrences of C. *difficile* infection, it has been unclear whether the high clinical treatment failure rate (up to 36%) was due to relapses or re-infections.[3] A recent study documented differing C. *difficile* DNA fingerprints in 15 out of 27 infected patients. Hence, at least 56% of the clinical recurrences of infection were due to re-infection as opposed to relapse.[14] An endemic C. *difficile* clone was present in 18 of the 27 studied patients (67%), accounting for 53% (31/58) of all isolates. It is, therefore,

Highlights in **Clostridium difficile** infection in practice *1997*

WHAT'S IN ?

- Increasing burden of C. *difficile* infection on healthcare resources
- Re-infections as opposed to relapses

WHAT'S OUT/GOING OUT ?

- Vancomycin for first-line treatment
- Routine examination of faecal specimens from patients with hospital-acquired diarrhoea for non-C. *difficile* causes

WHAT'S STILL CONTROVERSIAL ?

- Metronidazole resistance in C. *difficile*
- Biotherapeutic options for treatment
- Vaccination and other immunological approaches to treatment and prevention
- Environmental decontamination

likely that the majority of symptomatic recurrences were re-infections with either a different or the same C. *difficile* strain. These findings confirm those of two smaller studies,[15,16] and are consistent with recent results showing that sequential symptomatic episodes of C. *difficile* infection were not associated with increased disease severity.[17] Experimental treatment regimens have often been used for patients with multiple symptomatic episodes, but it is now clear that many such cases are re-infections as opposed to relapses.

Prophylaxis

Theoretically, vaccination against C. *difficile* toxin(s) or other antigens, particularly in high-risk individuals, could prevent infection. In a recent study, a plasmid containing DNA coding for amino acid residues from the non-toxic, receptor-binding moiety of C. *difficile* toxin A, was introduced into *Vibrio cholerae*, which was then administered orally to rabbits.[18] Colonization studies showed that the *V. cholerae* vector was recoverable from rabbit ilea for up to 5 days after oral inoculation, and systemic anti-C. *difficile* toxin A immunoglobulin G antibody responses were observed. Vaccination also led to significant protection against C. *difficile* toxin A in an ileal loop assay. The challenge remains to produce a vaccine that is efficacious in elderly patients in whom antibody responses are often impaired.

References

1. Ho M, Yang D, Wyle FA, Mulligan ME. Increased incidence of *Clostridium difficile*-associated diarrhea following decreased restriction of antibiotic use. *Clin Infect Dis* 1997;23(Suppl 1): S102–6.

2. *Clostridum difficile*: in England and Wales: quarterly report. *Commun Dis Rep CDR Wkly* 1997;7:412.

3. Wilcox MH, Cunniffe JG, Trundle C, Redpath C. Financial burden of hospital-acquired *Clostridum difficile* infection. *J Hosp Infect* 1996;34:23–30.

4. MacGowan AP, Feeney R, Brown I, McCulloch SY, Reeves DS, Lovering AM. Health care utilisation and antimicrobial use in elderly patients with community-acquired lower respiratory tract infection who develop *Clostridium difficile*-associated diarrhoea. *J Antimicrob Chemother* 1997;39: 537–41.

5. Starr JM, Rogers TR, Impallomeni M. Hospital-acquired *Clostridium difficile* diarrhoea and herd immunity. *Lancet* 1997;349:426–8.

6. Rohner P, Pittet D, Pepey B, Nije-Kinge T, Auckenthaler R. Etiological agents of infectious diarrhea: implications for requests for microbial culture. *J Clin Microbiol* 1997;35: 1427–32.

7. Pelaez T, Gijon P, Martinez L, Catalan P, Rivera ML, Bouza E. *Clostridium difficile* associated diarrhea in the AIDS era. Abstracts of the 37th Interscience Conference on Antimicrobial Agents and Chemotherapy. Toronto 1997. Abstract C28.

8. Wenisch C, Parschalk B, Hasenhundl M, Hirschl AM, Graninger W. Comparison of vancomycin, teicoplanin, metronidazole, and fusidic acid for the treatment of *Clostridium difficile*-associated diarrhea. *Clin Infect Dis* 1996;22:813–18.

9. Kelly CP, Pothoulakis C, Vavva F *et al*. Anti-C. *difficile* bovine immunoglobulin concentrate inhibits cytotoxicity and enterotoxicity of C. *difficile* toxins. *Antimicrob Agents Chemother* 1996; 40:373–9.

10. Kelly CP, Chetham S, Keates S *et al.* Survival of anti-C. *difficile* bovine immunoglobulin concentrate in the human gastrointestinal tract. *Antimicrob Agents Chemother* 1997;41:236–41.

11. Salcedo J, Keates S, Pothoulakis C *et al.* Intravenous immunoglobulin therapy for severe *Clostridium difficile* colitis. *Gut* 1997;41:366–70.

12. Johnson S. Antibody responses to clostridial infection in humans. *Clin Infect Dis* 1997;25(Suppl 2):S173–7.

13. Ward PB, Young GP. Dynamics of *Clostridium difficile* infection – control using diet. *Adv Exp Med Biol* 1997;412: 63–75.

14. Wilcox MH, Fawley WN, Settle CD, Davidson A. Recurrence of symptoms in *Clostridium difficile* infection – relapse or reinfection? *J Hosp Infect* 1998: In press.

15. Johnson S, Adelmann A, Clabots CR, Peterson LR, Gerding DN. Recurrences of *Clostridium difficile* diarrhea not caused by the original infecting organism. *J Infect Dis* 1989; 159:340–3.

16. O'Neill GL, Beaman MH, Riley TV. Relapse versus reinfection with *Clostridium difficile*. *Epidemiol Infect* 1991;107:627–35.

17. Fekety R, McFarland LV, Surawicz CM, Greenberg RN, Elmer GW, Mulligan ME. Recurrent *Clostridium difficile* diarrhea: characteristics of and risk factors for patients enrolled in a prospective, randomized, double-blinded trial. *Clin Infect Dis* 1997;24:324–33.

18. Ryan ET, Butterton JR, Smith RN, Carroll PA, Crean TI, Calderwood SB. Protective immunity against *Clostridium difficile* toxin A induced by oral immunization with a live, attenuated *Vibrio cholerae* vector strain. *Infect Immun* 1997;65:2941–9.

Hepatitis C infection

K Whitby and JA Garson

Department of Virology, University College London Medical School, London, UK

Progress in the diagnosis of hepatitis C virus (HCV) infection has been rapid since its discovery in 1989,[1] with increasing sensitivity and specificity of both serological and nucleic acid detection technologies. Over the same period the treatment of chronic HCV infection has largely, but not exclusively, been limited to the use of interferon alpha (IFNα). In this brief review we describe some of the most significant advances made in the field of HCV research over the past 12 months.

Development of proteinase inhibitors

Following the recent introduction of proteinase inhibitors for HIV-1 therapy,[2] efforts to develop similar treatment strategies for HCV have been vigorously pursued. The serine proteinase encoded by HCV non-structural gene 3 (NS3) is responsible for the post-translational cleavage of the viral polyprotein at four sites, and it is considered essential for virus replication. Soluble proteinases can be generated as 20 kDa N-terminal fragments of the 70 kDa NS3 protein using standard methods for recombinant protein expression. These fragments form the basis of many of the high throughput screening assays used by pharmaceutical companies to identify potential inhibitors. Chemical modification of the inhibitors thus identified can result in improved potency, reduced toxicity and increased bioavailability.

Love *et al.* have solved the X-ray structure of the NS3 proteinase domain at 2.4 Å resolution.[3] NS3 appears to be a zinc-containing metallo-proteinase with a catalytic triad of His-57, Asp-81 and Ser-139. Somewhat surprisingly, Love *et al.* observed that the Asp-81 side chain was oriented away from His-57, despite the fact that this would be expected to reduce the stability of the active site.

Simultaneous publication of the crystal structure of NS3 complexed with a synthetic NS4a peptide, showed that NS4a forms an integral part of the proteinase structure.[4] The structural anomalies reported by Love *et al.*, could simply be an artefact of crystallization, but would be more conveniently

Highlights in **Hepatitis C infection** *1997*

WHAT'S IN ?

- Combination antiviral therapy
- Development of proteinase inhibitors using 'rational drug design'
- HCV genome detection in pooled plasma products

WHAT'S OUT ?

- Ribavirin monotherapy

explained by the absence of NS4a. A noncovalent complex of these two intricately associated viral proteins may thus represent a second target for antiviral compounds.[5]

These findings will accelerate efforts to develop better anti-HCV agents via 'rational drug design' strategies.[6] However, progress in this area of HCV research is still hampered by the lack of an efficient *in-vitro* replication system.

Combination therapy

IFNα is currently the only licensed therapy for HCV infection. Unfortunately, virological and biochemical response is seen in only half of the patients treated, and only 15–20% sustain a response for more than 6 months post-therapy.[7] Attempts to increase the response rate have included:

- optimization of the dose and duration of therapy
- re-treatment of treatment failures
- use of the nucleoside analogue ribavirin in combination with IFNα.

In 1994 Brillanti *et al*. published a pilot study of IFNα plus ribavirin in patients who had previously failed to respond to IFNα monotherapy.[8] They reported that HCV-RNA became undetectable during therapy, and remained so for at least 6 months following therapy, in 40% of the patients. Since then, several groups have reported results from similar small, single centre studies confirming these findings.[9-11]

Earlier this year Schalm *et al.* published a meta-analysis of data from four trials of combination therapy at centres within Europe.[12] Three were randomized controlled trials and the fourth was an open study. In total, data from 186 patients, 78 of whom had received IFNα and ribavirin in combination, were included in the analysis. The estimated probability of a sustained virological and biochemical response in patients previously untreated with IFNα was 50%, and was similar in patients who had previously responded to IFNα monotherapy but relapsed. Of the patients who had failed to produce any response to previous IFNα monotherapy, 19% had cleared HCV-RNA from their serum at the end of therapy and remained negative for at least 6 months post therapy. The results of this meta-analysis reinforce the view that treatment with IFNα plus ribavirin represents a significant advance in the treatment of HCV infection.

Nucleic acid testing of pooled plasma products

Serological (i.e. antibody) screening of blood donations has helped to reduce the number of HCV-contaminated units entering the blood supply dramatically. However, occasional incidents of blood-product-related viral infection still occur,[13] and this is frequently due to the use of blood from donors in the seronegative 'window period'. The risk of infection increases with the number of units transfused, so a higher risk is associated with the use of products manufactured from pooled human plasma.

In an attempt to reduce the risk of acquiring HCV infection through the use of blood products further, regulations will soon be introduced requiring that plasma pools be tested for HCV-RNA. The sensitivity of the genome detection techniques employed for this purpose will clearly be critical. Viraemia levels encountered in HCV-infected individuals generally lie within the range 10^3–10^8 genomes/ml, with 10^6 being the approximate modal value.[14] Plasma pools may contain up to 20,000 donations, so that the final concentration of HCV-RNA in a pool containing a single HCV contaminated donation would be approximately 10^2 genomes/ml. Unfortunately, the lower detection limit of many genome amplification methods is around 10^3 genomes/ml, so that a proportion of contaminated pools may be missed. Efforts to enhance the sensitivity of polymerase chain reaction (PCR) systems to be able to detect such low level contamination are underway and a quantitative PCR assay with a detection limit of 40 genomes/ml has recently been described.[15] The increase in sensitivity afforded by this and similar systems should significantly increase the proportion of infected plasma pools detected. It is expected that progress and technical harmonization in this area will be greatly facilitated by the introduction of the WHO International HCV-RNA Standard.

References

1. Choo QL, Kuo G, Weiner AJ, Overby LR, Bradley DW, Houghton M. Isolation of a cDNA clone derived from a blood-borne non-A, non-B viral hepatitis genome. *Science* 1989;244:359–62.

2. Carpenter CC, Fischl MA, Hammer SM *et al*. Antiretroviral therapy for HIV infection in 1997. Updated recommendations of the International AIDS Society-USA panel. *JAMA* 1997;277(24):1962–9.

3. Love RA, Parge HE, Wickersham JA *et al*. The crystal structure of hepatitis C virus NS3 proteinase reveals a trypsin-like fold and a structural zinc binding site. *Cell* 1996;87:331–42.

4. Kim JL, Morgenstern KA, Lin C *et al*. Crystal structure of the hepatitis C virus NS3 protease domain complexed with a synthetic NS4a cofactor peptide. *Cell* 1996;87:343–55.

5. Clarke BE. Approaches to the development of novel inhibitors of hepatitis C virus replication. *J Viral Hepatitis* 1995;2:1–8.

6. Blundell TL. Structure-based drug design. *Nature* 1996;384(Suppl):23–6.

7. Jouet P, Roudot-Thorval F, Dhumeaux D, Metreau JM. Comparative efficacy of interferon-alpha in cirrhotic and noncirrhotic patients with non-A, non-B, C hepatitis. *Gastroenterology* 1994;106:686–90.

8. Brillanti S, Garson J, Foli M *et al*. A pilot study of combination therapy with ribavirin plus interferon alfa for interferon alfa-resistant chronic hepatitis C. *Gastroenterology* 1994;107:812–17.

9. Braconier JH, Paulsen O, Engman K, Widell A. Combined alpha interferon and ribavirin treatment in chronic hepatitis C: a pilot study. *Scand J Infect Disease* 1995;27:325–9.

10. Schvarcz R, Ando Y, Sönnerborg A, Weiland O. Combination treatment with interferon alpha-2b and ribavirin for chronic hepatitis C in patients who have failed to achieve sustained response to interferon alone: Swedish experience. *J Hepatol* 1995;23:17–21.

11. Telfer PT, Garson JA, Whitby K *et al*. Combination therapy with interferon alpha and ribavirin for chronic hepatitis C virus infection in thalassaemic patients. *Brit J Haematol* 1997;98:850–5.

12. Schalm SW, Hansen BE, Chemello L *et al*. Ribavirin enhances the efficacy but not the adverse effects of interferon in chronic hepatitis C. Meta-analysis of individual patient data from European centres. *J Hepatol* 1997;26(5):961–6.

13. Gomperts ED. HCV and Gammaguard in France. *Lancet* 1994;344:201.

14. Brillanti S, Garson JA, Tuke PW *et al*. Effect of α-interferon therapy on hepatitis C viraemia in community-acquired chronic non-A, non-B hepatitis: A quantitative polymerase chain reaction study. *J Med Virol* 1991;34:136–41.

15. Whitby K, Garson JA. A single tube two compartment reverse transcription polymerase chain reaction system for ultrasensitive quantitative detection of hepatitis C virus RNA. *J Virol Methods* 1997;66:15–18.

Viral infections in neutropenia

P Ljungman

Department of Hematology, Huddinge University Hospital, Karolinska Institute,
Huddinge, Sweden

Viral infections have long been recognized as major causes of morbidity and
mortality in patients undergoing allogeneic stem cell transplantation, but are
considered of minor importance compared with bacterial and fungal
infections in the neutropenic non-transplanted patient. Physicians, however,
need to be aware of changes in this field, particularly regarding respiratory
infections in the latter patient group. Recent developments regarding
infections with cytomegalovirus (CMV), human herpesvirus 6 (HHV-6),
respiratory viruses and the newly discovered hepatitis G virus (HGV) in
neutropenic patients and in those who have undergone allogeneic bone
marrow transplantation, are described here.

Herpesvirus infections

Cytomegalovirus. Despite early optimism, CMV disease still has a poor
prognosis in allogeneic bone marrow transplant recipients in 1997. In
particular, patients receiving transplants from unrelated bone marrow
donors have an increased risk for CMV disease.[1] It is now recognized that
CMV disease also occurs at various time spans after bone marrow
transplantation. Limaye *et al.* showed that, although rare, CMV disease
occurring before engraftment has a poor prognosis.[2] Furthermore, late CMV
disease occurring after day 100 is common, particularly after unrelated
donor transplantation, and correlates with a deficient specific T-cell response
to CMV.[3] Different strategies for disease prevention are available and must
be adapted to the individual patient. These strategies include prophylaxis
with antiviral agents or immunoglobulins, and pre-emptive therapy based on
sensitive diagnostic tests able to diagnose CMV infection before the disease
develops.

Anti-CMV hyperimmune globulin. Ruutu *et al.* performed a study aimed
at preventing primary CMV infection in seronegative marrow recipients
following CMV transmission from seropositive donors, using anti-CMV

hyperimmune globulin.[4] The study, however, showed no advantages with hyperimmune globulin in terms of preventing primary infection or CMV disease, or survival.

Acyclovir was the first antiviral agent to show efficacy in preventing CMV disease in bone marrow transplant recipients, and this was confirmed in a large study by Prentice *et al.* in 1994. Long-term follow-up data from this trial show that the positive effects on CMV viraemia and survival are maintained after prophylaxis is discontinued.[5]

Pre-emptive therapy. Boeckh *et al.* compared several different diagnostic tests and showed that the most sensitive was leukocyte-based polymerase chain reaction (PCR) followed by antigenaemia (pp-65 detection), plasma PCR, and viral culture.[6] The median number of days to the first positive test were 32, 42, 45 and 51 days, respectively. Woo *et al.* compared leukocyte-based and plasma-based PCR and concluded that leukocyte-based PCR was superior for guiding pre-emptive antiviral therapy.[7]

CMV disease is less frequent in autologous stem cell transplant recipients. Hebart *et al.* used leukocyte-based PCR to screen patients and showed that CMV-DNA was commonly detected after autologous stem cell transplantation, but its predictive value for CMV disease was low.[8] None of 98 patients undergoing autologous stem cell transplantation died from CMV disease and its incidence was rare. The low mortality risk associated with CMV disease is probably explained by the fact that most autologous stem cell transplant patients develop specific, protective, cell-mediated immunity within 100 days following transplantation.[9]

Human herpesvirus 6 (HHV-6) has several characteristics similar to CMV. Two different studies have shown that HHV-6 can often be detected after bone marrow transplantation.[10,11] The symptoms associated with HHV-6 infections in immunocompromised patients include encephalitis, bone marrow suppression, and pneumonia. Further studies are needed to establish the frequency of severe HHV-6 infections and current knowledge about therapy of HHV-6 disease is limited.

Respiratory virus infections

Respiratory syncytial virus (RSV) is a common infection both in infants, in whom it causes severe and sometimes life-threatening infections, and in

Highlights in **Viral infections in neutropenia** *1997*

WHAT'S IN ?

Cytomegalovirus

- Pre-emptive therapy with antiviral drugs
- PCR tests to guide pre-emptive therapy
- Antigenaemia

Respiratory viruses

- Important cause of morbidity and mortality in immunocompromised patients
- Infection control

WHAT'S OUT ?

Cytomegalovirus

- Immunoglobulins as prophylaxis
- Rapid isolation (DEAFF) for early diagnosis in bone marrow transplant patients

Hepatitis G virus

- Not important for liver disease in neutropenic patient

WHAT'S STILL CONTROVERSIAL ?

- Treatment of respiratory virus infections

healthy adults, in whom it causes mild upper respiratory symptoms. Recurrent infections are common throughout life. Over the last few years, RSV infections have emerged as severe threats in immunocompromised patients. Whimbey *et al.* have reported high mortality in RSV infection, both after allogeneic bone marrow transplantation and in patients treated for acute leukaemia.[12]

At present, it is unclear whether there is an effective treatment for RSV pneumonia. No controlled trials have been performed, although Whimbey *et al.* reported encouraging results with aerosolized ribavirin combined with immunoglobulin, which was associated with high anti-RSV titres.[12] Such treatment must be administered early before patients enter respiratory failure. Lewinsohn *et al.* and Sparrelid *et al.*, however, reported contradictory results from two small series of patients treated with intravenous ribavirin.[13,14] Thus, new strategies are needed in RSV infections. One option is early therapy for upper respiratory symptoms and another is infection containment, as RSV infections are often acquired and spread in hospitals. Garcia *et al.* showed that a combination of preventive strategies could significantly reduce the risk for nosocomial spread of RSV infection.[15]

Parainfluenza virus infections have several similarities to RSV infections in immunocompromised patients. Lewis *et al.* showed that 44% of bone marrow transplant patients infected with parainfluenza virus developed pneumonia, with an associated mortality of 37%.[16] The subtype of parainfluenza virus associated with highest morbidity and mortality seems to be type 3. No treatment studies have been published, but ribavirin has been administered as an aerosol and intravenously.[14,16] As with RSV infections, control of nosocomial spread is probably important for parainfluenza virus infections.

Hepatitis

Recently, HGV has been described. It is a flavivirus similar to hepatitis C virus and can be transmitted parenterally. Thus, patients with acute leukaemia and those undergoing stem cell transplantation are likely to become infected from the large number of blood transfusions that they receive. Two recently published studies have assessed the importance of HGV infection for liver complications in acute leukaemia and bone marrow transplant patients. In a study from Birmingham, UK, 48% of multitransfused patients with haematological malignancies were infected with HGV.[17] However, no association between HGV infection and liver function abnormalities could be found. In a study from Spain, HGV was found in 42% of allogeneic bone marrow transplant patients studied before and after transplantation.[18] This study also failed to establish any link between HGV infection and liver disease. Thus, it seems likely that this virus is of limited importance in multitransfused patients with haematological malignancies.

References

1. Takenaka K, Gondo H, Tanimoto K *et al*. Increased incidence of cytomegalovirus (CMV) infection and CMV-associated disease after allogeneic bone marrow transplantation from unrelated donors. The Fukuoka Bone Marrow Transplantation Group. *Bone Marrow Transplant* 1997;19:241–8.

2. Limaye A, Bowden R, Myerson D *et al*. Cytomegalovirus disease occurring before engraftment in marrow transplant recipients. *Clin Infect Dis* 1997;24: 830–5.

3. Krause H, Hebart H, Jahn G *et al*. Screening for CMV-specific T cell proliferation to identify patients at risk of developing late onset CMV disease. *Bone Marrow Transplant* 1997;19: 1111–16.

4. Ruutu T, Ljungman P, Brinch L *et al*. No prevention of cytomegalovirus infection by anti-cytomegalovirus hyperimmune globulin in seronegative bone marrow transplant recipients. *Bone Marrow Transplant* 1997;19:233–6.

5. Prentice H, Gluckman E, Powles R *et al*. Long-term survival in allogeneic bone marrow transplant recipients following acyclovir prophylaxis for CMV infection. The European Acyclovir for CMV Prophylaxis Study Group. *Bone Marrow Transplant* 1997;19: 129–33.

6. Boeckh M, Gallez-Hawkins G, Myerson D *et al*. Plasma polymerase chain reaction for cytomegalovirus DNA after allogeneic marrow transplantation: comparison with polymerase chain reaction using peripheral blood leukocytes, pp65 antigenemia, and viral culture. *Transplantation* 1997;64: 108–13.

7. Woo P, Lo S, Yuen K *et al*. Detection of CMV DNA in bone marrow transplant recipient: plasma versus leukocyte polymerase chain reaction. *J Clin Pathol* 1997;50:231–5.

8. Hebart H, Schroeder A, Löffler J *et al*. Cytomegalovirus monitoring by polymerase chain reaction of whole blood samples from patients undergoing autologous bone marrow or peripheral progenitor cell transplantation. *J Infect Dis* 1997;175:1490–3.

9. Reusser P, Attenhofer R, Hebart H *et al*. Cytomegalovirus-specific T-cell immunity in recipients of autologous peripheral blood stem cell or bone marrow transplants. *Blood* 1997;89: 3873–9.

10. Kadakia M, Rybka W, Stewart J *et al*. Human herpesvirus 6: infection and disease following autologous and allogeneic bone marrow transplantation. *Blood* 1996;87:5341–54.

11. Wang FZ, Dahl H, Linde A *et al*. Lymphotropic herpesviruses in allogeneic bone marrow transplantation. *Blood* 1996;88:3615–20.

12. Whimbey E, Englund J, Couch R. Community respiratory virus infections in immunocompromised patients with cancer. *Am J Med* 1997;102(3A):10–18.

13. Lewinsohn D, Bowden R, Matsson D *et al*. Phase I study of intravenous ribavirin treatment of respiratory syncytial virus pneumonia after marrow transplantation. *Antimicrob Agents Chemother* 1996;40:2555–7.

14. Sparrelid E, Ljungman P, Ekelöf-Andström E *et al*. Ribavirin therapy in bone marrow transplant recipients with viral respiratory tract infections. *Bone Marrow Transplant* 1997;19:905–8.

15. Garcia R, Raad I, Abi-Said D *et al*. Nosocomial respiratory syncytial virus infection: prevention and control in bone marrow transplant patients. *Infect Control Hosp Epidemiol* 1997;18:412–16.

16. Lewis V, Champlin R, Englund J *et al*. Respiratory disease due to parainfluenza virus in adult bone marrow transplant recipients. *Clin Infect Dis* 1996;23:1033–7.

17. Skidmore S, Collingham K, Harrison P *et al*. High prevalence of hepatitis G virus in bone marrow transplant recipients and patients treated for acute leukemia. *Blood* 1997;89:3853–6.

18. Rodriguez-Inigo E, Tomás J-F, Gomez-Garcia de Soria V *et al*. Hepatitis C and G virus infection and liver dysfunction after allogeneic bone marrow transplantation: results from a prospective study. *Blood* 1997;90:1326–31.

BSE and man

RW Lacey
Department of Microbiology, Chapel Allerton Hospital, Leeds, UK

Although a non-infectious aetiology for bovine spongiform encephalopathy (BSE), such as exposure to organophosphates, has been proposed, the transmission of the disease under farm and experimental conditions has established an infective basis for this and similar diseases in other species. Together, these diseases are properly described as transmissible spongiform encephalopathies (TSEs). Much of the early epidemiological and experimental research was performed on TSE in sheep (scrapie), sometimes after establishment of the infection in rodents. In general, TSEs can be transferred by the routes shown in Table 1, although the strength of the evidence varies.[1-7]

Nature of the infectious agent

The distinguishing characteristics of TSE – the spongiform encephalopathy – are microscopic vacuoles, loss of neurones, astrocytosis, and strands of polymeric proteins. The detailed elucidation of the infectious particle's chemical structure is slow because most means of characterizing micro-organisms (i.e. *in-vitro* culture and microscopy) are inappropriate. Furthermore, detection of the agent is not easy as it generally does not provoke an immune response and it does not contain nucleic acid. The presence of the particle is implied from animal transmission studies, but these are unsatisfactory in two important aspects:[1]

- the experiments are lengthy, varying from 6 months in rodents to several years in other long-lived animals and it is possible that disease only manifests itself after passage through more than one member of a species
- the nature of the infective agent changes unpredictably on interspecies transfer.

The prion hypothesis

In 1982, largely based on the agent's phenomenal resistance of infectivity to heat and irradiation, Prusiner suggested that it contained neither DNA nor

45

RNA but was proteinaceous (i.e. a prion) and could somehow catalyse its own synthesis.[8] All infectious agents must be able to replicate, and it is now known that prions use host genes,[9] which are referred to as *PrP* genes. The function of the general cellular protein (PrP) formed is uncertain, although animals devoid of it seem healthy. Although the normal PrP protein has been referred to as a prion, this term may be best used for the putative variant of the protein, PrP[sc], which is thought to be the infectious agent.

The origins of BSE

Despite claims to the contrary, the first BSE case was accurately identified in 1985. Following identification, 180,000 cases have been reported in the UK. The real number is probably 500,000 or more because many animals were slaughtered before they developed clinical disease, which appears on average at about 5 years. To date, the reported number of BSE cases in the rest of Europe is about 550. Again, the actual number is thought to be greater, but there is little evidence against BSE being a novel infection that originated in the UK. Since 1986, TSEs have been reported to occur spontaneously for the first time in 12 other mammals, including domestic cats and zoo species, in the UK. At London Zoo, 6 out of 14 greater kudu (African antelopes) have contracted TSE with evidence of acquisition from feed or vertical and/or horizontal transmission.

Because sporadic human infectious diseases are often acquired from animals (e.g. that due to *Salmonella enteritidis*), the source of sporadic Creutzfeldt-Jakob disease (CJD) is thought to be bovine, as sheep scrapie appears not to be responsible.[1] Sporadic CJD is associated with previous consumption of bovine products,[10] and the greater than expected number of cattle farmers contracting the disease supports this association.[11] If this is correct, the prevalence of TSE(s) in cattle decades ago must have gone undetected, and was presumably rare.

As a result of meat and bonemeal derived from cattle carcasses recycled back to cattle, BSE may be a new variant (nv) TSE, which almost certainly causes nvCJD. This hypothesis has ominous implications for the spread of nvCJD in the human population.

The species barrier

Experiments with varying doses and incubation periods have induced

Highlights in **BSE** in 1997

WHAT'S IN ?

- BSE can infect many species
- BSE has been spread between cattle by routes other than feed
- BSE is caused by a proteinaceous variant of a normal cell protein

WHAT'S OUT/GOING OUT ?

- BSE was not caused by sheep scrapie
- BSE was not caused by exposure to organophosphates

WHAT'S STILL CONTROVERSIAL ?

- The number of human cases of nvCJD acquired by direct transmission from cattle
- The potential for human-to-human spread of nvCJD via blood products, during surgery and vertically
- The handling of BSE by the UK government
- The prospect of relaxing the international ban on UK bovine material

uncertainty as to how readily a TSE can pass from one species to another.[1] However, once the infection has been established in a novel species, subsequent transfer within that species occurs readily; a low dose of the infectious agent can then cause the disease, possibly in a relatively short interval. Thus, transmission of sporadic CJD in the human population can occur within 3–5 years following administration of growth hormone[5] or blood transfusion,[6] although with the former the disease may take more than 15 years to appear.

The evidence that nvCJD is identical to BSE is based on similar clinical features in the two species, similar histological brain findings and a characteristic protein profile following Western blot analysis.[12] The unusually young ages of nvCJD patients and BSE cattle also support a common identity of the infection and has disturbing implications for human health. With TSEs in general, many tissues are capable of transmitting infection at around a third to half of the time before symptoms are apparent.[1] The cells of the reticulo-endothelial system provide the means for the initial prion replication, which is why in 1989 specific bovine offals, including the spleen, thymus, tonsils and intestines, were banned.

The threat

Thus, while the potential for spread of BSE to man is grave in itself, the subsequent spread within the human population could be disastrous. By analogy with HIV, and with our understanding of TSEs in general, the potential routes of transfer include maternal transmission,[7] blood transfusion,[6] surgical instruments, transplants and intravenous drug abuse (Table 1). Unlike HIV, however, there is no validated predictive test to identify subclinical carriers and no available drug treatment.

TABLE 1

Routes of TSE acquisition	Strength of evidence
Food	+ + +
Injection (contaminated growth hormone, blood, grafts, transplants)	+ + +
Lateral (sheep, goats, rodents)	+ +
Environment (sheep in Iceland)	+ +
Vertical (prior to birth)	+ + +
Breast secretions	+ +
Seminal fluid	+

+ + + near certainty
+ + probable
+ possible

References

1. Dealler SF, Lacey RW. Transmissible spongiform encephalopathies: the threat of BSE to man. *Food Microbiol* 1990;7: 253–79.

2. Pattison IH. The spread of scrapie by contact between affected and healthy sheep, goats or mice. *Vet Rec* 1964;76: 333–6.

3. Dickinson AG, Mackay JMK, Zlotnik I. Transmission by contact of scrapie in mice. *J Comp Pathol* 1964;74: 250–6.

4. Pattison IH, Hoare MN, Jeffett JN, WatsonWA. Spread of scrapie to sheep and goats by oral dosing with focal membranes from scrapie-affected sheep. *Vet Rec* 1972;90:465–8.

5. Brown P, Preece MA, Will RG. "Friendly fire" in medicine: hormones, homo-grafts and Creutzfeldt-Jakob disease. *Lancet* 1992;340:24–7.

6. Klein R, Dumble LJ. Transmission of Creutzfeld-Jakob disease. *Lancet* 1993;341:768.

7. Lacey RW, Dealler SF. Vertical transfer of prion disease. *Hum Reprod* 1994;9:1792–6.

8. Prusiner SB. Novel proteinaceous infection particles cause sheep scrapie. *Science* 1982;216:136–44.

9. Bueler H, Aguzzi A, Saiter A *et al*. Mice devoid of PrP are resistant to scrapie. *Cell* 1993;73:1339–47.

10. Annual reports of the Creutzfeldt-Jakob Surveillance Unit, Edinburgh 1994, 1997. Department of Health.

11. Consero SN, Zeidler M, Esmonde TF *et al*. Sporadic Creutzfeldt-Jakob disease in the United Kingdom: analysis of epidemiological surveillance data for 1970–96. *BMJ* 1997;315:389–96.

12. Collinge J, Siddle KCL, Meads J, Ironside J, Hill AF. Molecular analysis of prion strain variation and the aetiology of 'new variant' CJD. *Nature* 1996;383: 685–90.

Glycopeptide-resistant enterococci

JE McGowan Jr

Rollins School of Public Health of Emory University, and Emory University School of Medicine, Atlanta, Georgia, USA

In the past year, glycopeptide-resistant enterococci (GRE) have been brought to greater public attention as a result of news reports about these 'untreatable' organisms. In many accounts, the organisms are referred to as 'vancomycin-resistant enterococci' (VRE), but should properly be called GRE, as most clinically relevant strains are resistant to teicoplanin, as well as other glycopeptide antimicrobials. Although substantial progress has recently been made in the epidemiology, diagnosis and prevention of infections due to GRE, few improvements in treatment have, however, emerged.

Occurrence

GRE strains now occur worldwide,[1] and are noteworthy for several reasons. GRE strains that were consistently susceptible to a combination of penicillins and aminoglycosides for decades have now developed resistance, not only to these classic agents, but to newer drugs as well. Indeed, GRE have developed resistance to recently introduced antimicrobials (e.g. fluoroquinolones) almost as soon as the drugs have been marketed. In addition, the number of GRE strains that are resistant to several different groups of antimicrobials has increased during the past few years. It has also been found that infections due to GRE that were formerly localized primarily in the intensive care units (ICU) of hospitals in the USA and in specialized areas, such as dialysis and liver units, in the UK, now occur in other in-patient, and even in ambulatory care, settings.[2–4]

Clinical and economic importance

Papers presented at recent meetings disagree about the impact of resistance in GRE on the clinical outcome of severe infections. A group in New York, USA, found no significant difference in crude mortality between bacteraemic patients with VRE and those infected with organisms susceptible to

Highlights in **Glycopeptide-resistant enterococci** 1997

WHAT'S IN ?

- Discovery of *van*D resistance mechanism
- Attempts at combination therapy to seek synergistic activity
- Clinical trials of new fluoroquinolones and dalfopristin/quinupristin
- Modified methods for detecting resistance by automated instruments
- Barrier isolation as the major technique for control of clonal spread in hospitals

WHAT'S OUT ?

- Enthusiasm for chloramphenicol

WHAT'S CONTROVERSIAL ?

- Impact of antimicrobial use in animals on spread of GRE in humans

vancomycin.[5] In contrast, a recent 2-year, prospective, multicentre study of 375 patients with enterococcal bacteraemia found that vancomycin resistance was a significant independent predictor of mortality.[6]

The economic impact of infections with GRE compared with those due to vancomycin-susceptible strains continues to be debated. A study in the USA found that patients with VRE spent twice as long in ICU compared with those infected with susceptible isolates (2.1 versus 1.1 days, respectively); however, the duration of antibiotic therapy, time to negative cultures, and underlying disease states were similar for both groups.[7] By contrast, another study found that VRE strains causing bloodstream infection were associated with a hospital stay of 26 days compared with 12 days for susceptible strains, after adjusting for patient type, administration of chemotherapy, gender, age and admission APACHE II score.[8] It appears, therefore, that a large multicentre study is required to resolve this issue.

Pathogenesis

A diversity of phenotypes characterizes GRE strains.[9] Three phenotypes were identified according to the antibacterial and resistance-inducing activity of vancomycin and teicoplanin. Now, however, a new phenotype has been described, *van*D, characterized by resistance to moderate concentrations of vancomycin and low level resistance (or even susceptibility) to teicoplanin.[10] The clinical impact of this newly recognized variant is unclear. However, its appearance signals a call to microbiologists to examine diagnostic methods to ensure that this new phenotype can be identified.

Epidemiology

Reports of multicentre studies dealing with risk determinants for GRE have now begun to appear. A comparison of infection with VRE and infection with vancomycin-susceptible enterococci at 20 hospitals in the USA over a 2-year period found significant differences between the two groups.[11] These included prior vancomycin use, anti-anaerobic agent use and presence of multiple underlying illnesses. Previous exposure to β-lactam drugs was not found to be an important factor. However, as rectal and skin colonization with VRE is common in patients who develop bacteraemia due to this organism,[12] this may increase the risk of catheter-related sepsis, cross-infection and contamination of specimens for blood culture.

The role of the hospital environment in transmission of GRE is now receiving more attention.[13] Admission to a hospital room recently occupied by a VRE-colonized patient has been identified as an independent risk factor for VRE colonization.[14]

Another environmental aspect is the use of antimicrobials in animal feeds.[15] Internationally, GRE can be found in foods and in the intestinal tracts of non-hospitalized persons, especially in areas where avoparcin (a glycopeptide used as a growth promoter) has been used in animal feeds.[1] A study from London, UK, however, concluded that VRE "from poultry and humans represent two distinct populations".[16] The topic therefore remains controversial.

Diagnosis

The emergence and dissemination of GRE has led to recommendations for updating both microbiological surveillance and clinical detection methods. A recent survey documents that diagnostic techniques generally have been modified so that they successfully recognize GRE in specimens from patients with clinical illness.[17] Rapid screening schemes now employ both phenotype-based and amplification techniques.[18] These hold the promise of efficient characterization of GRE strains within 24 hours.

Treatment

Few new treatment options have proven effective.[19] As GRE strains are typically resistant to multiple antimicrobial drugs, finding synergistic drug combinations is difficult.

Dalfopristin/quinupristin (Synercid) is effective *in vitro* against many GRE strains of *Enterococcus faecium* (it is not active against *E. faecalis*).[20] It has also been found to be effective in about three-quarters of reported cases of *E. faecium* infection in severely ill patients.[21] Both superinfection and resistance emerging during the course of therapy have been reported, but at low rates.[22]

Enthusiasm for use of chloramphenicol to treat strains susceptible in the laboratory has moderated as clinical experience has been accumulated. In some areas, most strains of GRE are also resistant to chloramphenicol and, even when the organism is susceptible *in vitro*, the evidence for successful clinical impact is slim.[23]

New approaches to therapy include combining β-lactam drugs with glycopeptides or fluoroquinolones. How useful these combinations will be remains to be seen; one study presented this year found no difference in clinical improvement between patients who received monotherapy and those who received combination treatment.[11] Newer fluoroquinolone drugs show greater *in-vitro* activity against GRE than earlier drugs of this group; however, the clinical relevance of this remains to be proven.[24]

Prevention

Control of GRE infections usually requires a combination of activities. Measures against cross-infection (primarily barrier isolation precautions) can be effective in reducing clonal spread.[13] For example, one hospital in Los

Angeles, USA, recently found that infection control measures were effective in limiting an institution-wide outbreak;[25] a similar experience was reported in a paediatric oncology unit in California, USA.[26] A study in Chicago, USA, however, found that more patients entered the ICU with VRE than acquired it while they were there. The authors suggested that control of many different classes of antimicrobials may be needed throughout their hospital, in addition to infection control compliance, if intervention is to be successful.[27]

Use of nonabsorbable antimicrobials has been suggested as a means for controlling spread of GRE. However, a recent report questions this approach. Oral bacitracin, 25,000 U every 6 hours orally in gel capsule form, had no effect on intestinal colonization of *E. faecalis* and was 'minimally effective' in reducing overall VRE stool colonization.[28]

In formulating control strategies and treatment guidelines, national or regional recommendations must be modified to take into account local features, problems and resources. For example, plans for the control of resistant strains of GRE in long-term care facilities must be customized to the patients and types of care given in these facilities.[29]

References

1. McDonald LC, Jarvis WR. The global impact of vancomycin-resistant enterococci. *Curr Opin Infect Dis* 1997; 10:304–9.

2. Boyce JM. Vancomycin-resistant enterococcus – detection, epidemiology, and control measures. *Infect Dis Clin N Am* 1997;11:367–84.

3. Morrison D, Cooke RPD, Kaufmann ME, Cookson BD, Stephenson J. Inter-hospital spread of vancomycin-resistant *Enterococcus faecium. J Hosp Infect* 1997;36:77–80.

4. Lavery A, Rossney AS, Morrison D, Power A, Keane CT. Incidence and detection of multi-drug resistant enterococci in Dublin hospitals. *J Med Microbiol* 1997;46:150–6.

5. Curbelo DE, Koll BS, Wilets I, Raucher B. Treatment and outcome in 100 patients with vancomycin resistant enterococcal bacteremia. Abstracts of the 37th Interscience Conference on Antimicrobial Agents and Chemotherapy, Toronto, Canada, Sept 30–Oct 3 1997:289(Abstract J-7).

6. Vergis EN, Chow JW, Haydn MK *et al*. Vancomycin resistance predicts mortality in enterococcal bacteremia: a prospective, multicenter study of 375 patients. Abstracts of the 37th Interscience Conference on Antimicrobial Agents and Chemotherapy, Toronto, Canada, Sept 30–Oct 3 1997:289 (Abstract J-6).

7. Jamali R, Lubowski TJ, Dever LL, O'Donovan CA. The economic impact of treating vancomycin-resistant enterococcus infections in a VA Medical Center. *Clin Infect Dis* 1997;25:420.

8. Montecalvo MA, Uman J, Petrullo C *et al*. The cost-benefit of enhanced infection control strategies to prevent transmission of vancomycin resistant enterococci. Abstracts of the 37th Interscience Conference on Antimicrobial Agents and Chemotherapy, Toronto, Canada, Sept 30–Oct 3 1997:303 (Abstract J-84).

9. Leclercq R, Courvalin P. Resistance to glycopeptides in enterococci. *Clin Infect Dis* 1997;24:545–56.

10. Perichon B, Reynolds P, Courvalin P. VanD-type glycopeptide-resistant *Enterococcus faecium* BM4339. *Antimicrob Agents Chemother* 1997;41:2016–8.

11. Bhavnani SM, Goudbourn JA, Deinhart JA, Jones RN, Ballow CH, National Nosocomial Resistance Surveillance Group. A nationwide, multicenter, case-control study comparing risk factors, treatment, and outcome for vancomycin-resistant and susceptible enterococcal bacteremia. Abstracts of the 37th Interscience Conference on Antimicrobial Agents and Chemotherapy, Toronto, Canada, Sept 30–Oct 3 1997:293(Abstract J-30).

12. Beezhold DW, Slaughter S, Hayden MK *et al*. Skin colonization with vancomycin-resistant enterococci among hospitalized patients with bacteremia. *Clin Infect Dis* 1997;24:704–6.

13. Weber DJ, Rutala WA. Role of environmental contamination in the transmission of vancomycin-resistant enterococci. *Infect Control Hosp Epidemiol* 1997;18:306–9.

14. Jernigan JA, Pullen A, Nolte FS, Patel P, Rimland D. The role of the hospital environment in nosocomial transmission of vancomycin resistant enterococci; a retrospective cohort study. Abstracts of the Infectious Disease Society of America 35th Annual Meeting, San Francisco, Sept 1997. *Clin Infect Dis* 1997;25:363 (Abstract 46).

15. Das I, Fraise A, Wise R. Are glycopeptide-resistant enterococci in animals a threat to human beings? *Lancet* 1997;349:997–8.

16. Kirk M, Beighton D, Chen HY, Hill R, Casewell MW. Phenotypic differentiation of human and poultry vancomycin-resistant *Enterococcus faecium*. Abstracts of the 37th Interscience Conference on Antimicrobial Agents and Chemotherapy, Toronto, Canada, Sept 30–Oct 3 1997:69 (Abstract C-135).

17. Endtz HP, Van den Braak N, Goessens WHF *et al*. Comparison of seven methods, including a new Vitek GPS-101 card, to detect vancomycin resistance in enterococci. Abstracts of the 37th Interscience Conference on Antimicrobial Agents and Chemotherapy, Toronto, Canada, Sept 30–Oct 3 1997:91(Abstract D-43).

18. Sahm DF, Free L, Smith C, Eveland M, Mundy LM. Rapid characterization schemes for surveillance isolates of vancomycin-resistant enterococci. *J Clin Microbiol* 1997;35:2026–30.

19. Landman D, Quale JM. Management of infections due to resistant enterococci: a review of therapeutic options. *J Antimicrob Chemother* 1997;40:161–70.

20. Evans PA, Norden CW, Rhoads S, Deobaldia J, Silber JL. *In vitro* susceptibilities of clinical isolates of vancomycin-resistant enterococci. *Antimicrob Agents Chemother* 1997; 41:1406.

21. Moellering RC Jr, Linden PK for the Synercid® Emergency-Use Study Group. Efficacy and safety of quinupristin/dalfopristin (Synercid®) in the treatment of vancomycin-resistant *Enterococcus faecium* (VREF) infections. 3rd International Conference on the Macrolides, Azalides and Streptogramins ; Lisbon, Portugal, 24–26 January 1997;Abstract.

22. Nadler H, Dowzicky M, Talbot G, Bompart F, Grote F. Low rates of emerging resistance and superinfection in Synercid (dalfopristin/quinupristin) treated patients. 4th International Conference on the Macrolides, Azalides, Streptogramins and Ketolides; Barcelona, Spain, 21–23 January 1998:Abstract 2.10.

23. Lautenbach E, Bilker WB, Schuster MG, Brennan PJ. Chloramphenicol in the treatment of vancomycin-resistant enterococcal bacteremia. Abstracts of the Infectious Disease Society of America Annual Meeting, San Francisco, Sept 1997. *Clin Infect Dis* 1997;25:435 (Abstract 433).

24. Martinez-Martinez L, Joyanes P, Pascual A, Terrero E, Perea EJ. Activity of eight fluoroquinolones against enterococci. *Clin Microbiol Infect* 1997;3:497–9.

25. Schneider S, Murthy R. Impact of infection control measures on a hospital outbreak with vancomycin-resistant *E. faecium*. Abstracts of the Infectious Diseases Society of America 35th Annual Meeting, San Francisco, Sept 1997. *Clin Infect Dis* 1997;25:425(Abstract 382).

26. Nourse C, Murphy H, Byrne C *et al*. Eradication of vancomycin-resistant *Enterococcus faecium* from a paediatric oncology unit and risk factors for colonisation of patients. Abstracts of the Infectious Diseases Society of America 35th Annual Meeting, San Francisco, Sept 1997. *Clin Infect Dis* 1997;24:419 (Abstract 344).

27. Fleenor-Ford A, Fridkin S, Pur S *et al*. Acquisition of vancomycin resistant enterococcus in a medical intensive care unit: analysis for risk factors amenable to intervention. Abstracts of the Infectious Disease Society of America 35th Annual Meeting, San Francisco, Sept 1997. *Clin Infect Dis* 1997;25:436(Abstract 435).

28. Montecalvo MA, Raffalli J, Rodney K, Petrullo C, Jarvis WR, Wormser GP. Effect of oral bacitracin on the number of vancomycin resistant enterococci in stool. Abstracts of the 37th Interscience Conference on Antimicrobial Agents and Chemotherapy, Toronto, Canada, Sept 30–Oct 3 1997:303(Abstract J-80).

29. Bonilla HF, Zervos MA, Lyons MJ *et al*. Colonization with vancomycin-resistant *Enterococcus faecium*: comparision of a long-term-care unit with an acute-care hospital. *Infect Control Hosp Epidemiol* 1997;18: 333–9.

Multiple-drug-resistant tuberculosis

F Drobniewski

Public Health Laboratory & Medical Microbiology, King's College School of Medicine & Dentistry, London, UK

Mycobacterium tuberculosis currently infects almost one-third of the world's population. Each year about 8 million new clinical cases occur leading to almost 3 million deaths.[1,2]

Drug resistance develops spontaneously in bacteria at a particular rate for a given drug. Non-adherence to therapy, inappropriate drug prescribing, malabsorption, poor quality drugs and deterioration of public health infrastructure needed for adequate supervision of treatment lead to selection of drug-resistant mutants and treatment failure. Drug-resistance trends in patients who have not previously received anti-tuberculosis (TB) drugs (primary or initial drug resistance) and in those who have been treated previously (acquired drug resistance) are crude indicators of the effectiveness of a national TB programme. High rates of multiple-drug-resistant TB (MDRTB) (i.e. resistance to isoniazid and rifampicin – two of the major first-line drugs) are indicative of poorly functioning programmes.[3–6] Recent dramatic outbreaks of MDRTB in the USA and Europe, particularly in HIV-infected patients, have focused attention on the emergence of drug resistance, its epidemiology, treatment and outcome.

Prominent outbreaks continued to be described in 1997 and molecular techniques, such as DNA fingerprinting, played an important role in defining transmission. For example, the first substantial outbreak of MDRTB due to *M. bovis* was reported in Madrid and involved 19 individuals in whom restriction fragment length polymorphism and spoligotyping (an amplification and hybridization technique) were used to identify transmission.[7] Strains were resistant to isoniazid, rifampicin, pyrazinamide (as are all *M. bovis* isolates), ethambutol, streptomycin, amikacin, para-aminosalicylic acid, clarithromycin, cycloserine, ofloxacin, capreomycin and ethionamide. In Buenos Aires from October to December 1996, over 300 patients were diagnosed with MDRTB isolates (in this case, involving resistance to isoniazid, rifampicin and up to four other drugs) possessing an indistinguishable DNA fingerprint.[8]

Epidemiology

The true current level of drug resistance in the world is unknown, although some studies and anecdotal evidence indicate that it has been increasing in recent years. Unfortunately, several methodological problems prevent a clear global picture developing. These include:

- the absence of adequate culture facilities
- the use of non-standardized methodologies
- the absence of quality-control measures
- the absence of longitudinal studies to detect trends
- the failure to differentiate between primary and acquired drug resistance
- the inherent selection bias of many surveys, particularly those centred on large cities and specialized hospitals.

Nevertheless, Cohn et al. have summarized the results from 63 representative surveys.[4] The prevalence ranges of primary drug resistance were 0–16.9% for isoniazid, 0–3% for rifampicin, 0–4.2% for ethambutol and 0.1–23.5% for streptomycin. The prevalences of acquired drug resistance for the same drugs were 4–53.7%, 0–14.5%, 0–13.7% and 0–19.4%, respectively. High levels of acquired MDRTB were noted in New York City, USA (30.1%), Bolivia (15.3%), Korea (14.5%), Gujarat, India (33.8%) and Nepal (48.0%).

In 1994, WHO and the International Union Against Tuberculosis and Lung Disease began the Global Project on Anti-tuberculosis Drug Resistance Surveillance, which reported the results of surveys and surveillance programmes from 35 countries.[6] The project was designed to measure drug prevalence using standardized methods guided by three overriding principles, that:

- the study sample of TB patients was representative of cases within the whole country
- laboratory performance was validated
- primary and acquired drug resistance could be distinguished.

A key part of the programme was the creation of a Global Network of Supranational Reference Laboratories (SRLs), currently located in 17 countries, to serve as reference centres for quality control of drug susceptibility testing in national surveys.[9]

In the 35 countries surveyed as part of the WHO programme, data on 50,000 patients sampled from 20% of the world's population were collated.

Highlights in **Multiple-drug-resistant tuberculosis 1997**

WHAT'S CONTROVERSIAL ?

Treatment

- Duration of therapy
- Role of rapid molecular investigations
- Role for rifamycins such as rifabutin and rifapentine

Vaccines

- Role of BCG
- *Mycobacterium vaccae*

All but three countries differentiated between primary (or initial) and acquired drug resistance. Overall agreement between the SRLs and national reference centres was 96%. Drug resistance was seen in all countries with a median prevalence of approximately 10% (range 2–41%) in new patients. MDRTB was widespread with a third of countries surveyed having levels above 2% in new patients; the median prevalence was 1.4% in new patients (range 0–14%), although very high rates were found in former countries of the USSR, the Baltic Republics, Argentina, India and China (Table 1).[6] In general, countries with poor national TB programmes had a higher prevalence of MDRTB. The successful implementation of standardized short-course chemotherapy (SSC) was associated with a lower level of drug resistance.

Other detailed trend analyses were published in 1997 in addition to those associated with the WHO programme. A recent study described drug-resistant TB rates in culture-positive cases from 1993 to 1996 in the USA.[10] Overall resistance was 8.4% to isoniazid and 3.0% to rifampicin, and MDRTB was 2.2% with resistance rates to pyrazinamide, streptomycin and ethambutol of 3.0%, 6.2% and 2.2%, respectively. A total of 1457 MDRTB cases were reported from 42 states, New York City and Washington DC, but 38% of cases came from New York City. MDRTB and rifampicin

TABLE 1

Prevalence of multiple-drug-resistant tuberculosis in 12 countries (1994–97)[6]

Country	Primary multiple-drug resistance (%)	Acquired multiple-drug resistance (%)	Combined multiple-drug resistance prevalence*
Argentina	4.6	22.2	8.0
Dominican Republic	6.6	19.7	8.6
Estonia	10.2	19.2	11.7
Ivory Coast	5.3	–	–
Latvia	14.4	54.4	22.1
Peru	2.5	15.7	4.5
Puerto Rico	1.9	13.6	2.6
Republic of Korea	1.6	27.5	3.1
Romania	2.8	14.4	3.6
Russia (Ivanovo Oblast)	4.0	27.3	7.3
USA	1.6	7.1	2.0
Zimbabwe	1.9	8.3	2.4

* Prevalence of drug resistance regardless of history of prior treatment[6]

mono-resistance rates were similar among US- and foreign-born patients. In patients born in the USA, drug resistance was significantly higher among those with HIV infection. Overall, MDRTB incidence decreased after 1991, although this was mainly due to the significant reduction in cases in New York City. Unfortunately, DNA fingerprinting has indicated that the highly drug-resistant strain that caused several large outbreaks in New York City in the 1990s has spread to nine states in the USA and Puerto Rico.[11]

In the UK, a surveillance system, MYCOBNET, was created as a laboratory-based surveillance system for antibiotic drug resistance in *M. tuberculosis*. Preliminary trend analysis for 1993–96 showed that initial MDRTB incidence rates increased from 0.6% to 1.2% and the combined clinical prevalence rate (the aggregate proportion of MDRTB cases in a given year) rose from 0.6 to 1.7%.[12]

Treatment of MDRTB

Since chemotherapy became possible in the 1940s and 1950s, the principles of treatment have not changed and include the use of combination chemotherapy in standardized regimens, usually for 6–9 months. WHO has emphasized the role of short-course, directly observed treatment as a key strategy in which drug administration is monitored by a healthcare worker. In a recent WHO study, national TB programmes adopting such a control strategy achieved higher cure rates than those that did not.[2] While this is important, both for ensuring the successful treatment of infectious cases and for the prevention of emerging drug resistance including MDRTB, the development of new drugs, vaccines and other control strategies should also be of high priority.[13]

Nevertheless, treatment of MDRTB cases is difficult, prolonged and associated with a high mortality rate, particularly in immunocompromised patients. Treatment should be determined with regard to the guidelines in Table 2.[3,5] In practice, in the developing world where the greatest burden of

---

TABLE 2

Guidelines for treating multiple-drug-resistant tuberculosis[3,5]

- Use drug susceptibility data to plan therapy
- Use at least three agents to which the organism is susceptible
- Include as many bactericidal agents as possible
- Never add a single agent to a failing regimen
- Use directly observed therapy
- Consider incentives to support therapy
- Consider any patient factors that might interfere with the choice or absorption of treatment

cases exists, standard treatment will be ineffective in MDRTB cases and second-line therapies are usually unavailable.

Although research has identified new targets to which novel drugs could be developed, in 1997 most new agents were derivatives of existing drugs, such as fluoroquinolones. Research into novel rifamycins has produced controversial results. Rifabutin has been used mostly for prophylaxis against *M. avium-intracellulare*, but is as effective against sensitive *M. tuberculosis* as rifampicin. Some rifampicin-resistant strains are sensitive to rifabutin, but rifabutin should only be used with clear documented sensitivity and in practice this is of limited use. In HIV-positive patients who are receiving some protease inhibitors, however, rifabutin may be a useful alternative to rifampicin as it causes less liver enzyme induction, although monitoring of both drug levels is usually required.[14] Its use has been associated previously with acquired rifampicin mono-resistance in a small number of HIV-positive patients when used for *M. avium-intracellulare* prophylaxis. Rifapentine, which has a long half-life, has been evaluated in clinical trials where it was given once weekly with daily isoniazid during the continuation phase. In a Hong Kong study, however, Chinese formulations with sub-optimal bioavailability produced high relapse rates.[14] An improved formulation is undergoing trials in the USA and South Africa although preliminary results in the USA trial have also indicated a high rate of relapse with acquired rifampicin mono-resistance.[14]

The use of *M. vaccae* as an immunotherapeutic adjunct to chemotherapy is also being evaluated in several locations in Europe, Asia and Africa. Despite some recent encouraging results from Romania,[15,16] disappointing results of a randomized controlled trial in Durban, South Africa have recently been reported.[17] Patients with TB-positive sputum smears were randomized to receive chemotherapy alone or chemotherapy with *M. vaccae* given at day 7 of treatment. The primary endpoint was sputum culture conversion in the first 8 weeks. It was hypothesized that *M. vaccae* would have a rapid effect on the immune system so that proportionally more patients receiving immunotherapy would convert to culture negativity. The proportion of patients converting to culture negativity and the survival rate at 8 weeks, however, were the same in each group. It is difficult to see how any adjunct therapy could improve on the conversion and cure rates obtained with optimal, directly observed chemotherapy in this time frame, and arguably a trial in patients with drug resistance might be more beneficial.

Published data on the use of immunomodulating cytokines in refractory TB are limited, but one recent small study indicated that there was some survival benefit when appropriate chemotherapy was augmented with aerosolized interferon-γ in patients with pulmonary disease.[18]

Diagnosis of MDRTB

Earlier studies in New York clearly indicated the importance, in terms of survival, of rapid diagnosis of MDRTB and the determination of drug susceptibility for individualized therapy. Culture-based techniques remain the basis of drug susceptibility testing and several studies employing novel automated rapid culture systems were published in 1997. Molecular detection of drug resistance in clinical laboratories has been facilitated by basic research, and the identification and sequencing of the *emb* genes responsible for most ethambutol resistance[19,20] has continued to develop our understanding of the mechanisms of resistance to anti-tuberculosis drugs.

In the UK, the Public Health Laboratory Service Mycobacterium Reference Unit has implemented a national molecular detection of rifampicin resistance service as part of a strategy to identify MDRTB isolates quickly, as 90% of rifampicin-resistant isolates are also resistant to isoniazid. In 1997, Nash *et al.* described a strategy using an RNA-RNA mismatch assay to identify rifampicin resistance,[21] and Wilson *et al.* described a novel phenotypic assay, PhaB, using mycobacteriophages for drug susceptibility testing.[22] Using the former assay on 46 isolates, the specificity and sensitivity for detecting rifampicin resistance was 100% and 96%, respectively. The PhaB assay correctly assigned rifampicin susceptibility in 44/46 (96%) of isolates within 2 days.

Conclusion

MDRTB continues to offer a challenge to clinicians, clinical microbiologists and epidemiologists, both in diagnosing cases and defining the scale of the problem. It challenges scientists to develop novel treatment strategies and vaccines that will continue to be needed if TB is to be conquered. TB is a disease that remains the most important single infectious cause of mortality in the world today.

References

1. Drobniewski F, Pablos-Mendez A, Raviglione MC. Epidemiology of tuberculosis in the world. *Semin Respir Med* 1997;18:419–29.

2. Raviglione MC, Dye C, Schmidt S, Kuchi A. The WHO Global Surveillance and Monitoring Project. Assessment of worldwide tuberculosis control. *Lancet* 1997;350:624–9.

3. Drobniewski FA. Is death inevitable with multiresistant TB plus HIV infection? *Lancet* 1997;349:71–2.

4. Cohn DL, Bustreo F, Raviglione MC. Drug-resistant tuberculosis: review of the worldwide situation and the WHO/IUATLD Global Surveillance Project. International Union against Tuberculosis and Lung Disease. *Clin Infect Dis* 1997;24(Suppl 1):S121–30.

5. Drobniewski F. Multiple drug resistance in the developed world. *Alpe Adria Microbiology J* 1997;1:15–21.

6. World Health Organisation/ International Union Against Tuberculosis and Lung Disease. Anti-tuberculosis drug resistance in the world. Geneva, Switzerland: WHO, 1997.

7. Blazquez J, Espinosa-de-los-Monteros LE, Samper S *et al.* Genetic characterization of multidrug resistant *Mycobacterium bovis* strains from a hospital outbreak involving human immunodeficiency virus positive patients. *J Clin Microbiol* 1997;35:1390–3.

8. Weinbaum C, Ridzon R, Joglar O *et al.* Multidrug resistant TB (MDRTB) among AIDS patients in an infectious disease hospital, Buenos Aires. *Int J Tuberc Lung Dis* 1997;1:S24.

9. Laszlo A, Rahman M, Raviglione M, Bustreo F, WHO/IUATLD Network of Supranational Reference Laboratories. Quality assurance programme for drug susceptibility testing of *Mycobacterium tuberculosis* in the WHO/IUATLD Supranational Laboratory Network: first round of proficiency testing. *Int J Tuberc Lung Dis* 1997;1:231–8.

10. Moore M, Onorato IM, McCray E, Castro KG. Trends in drug-resistant tuberculosis in the United States, 1993–1996. *JAMA* 1997;278:833–7.

11. Agerton T, Valway S, Onorato I. Spread of a highly drug resistant strain of *M. tuberculosis* (Strain W) in the United States. *Int J Tuberc Lung Dis* 1997; 1:S23.

12. Bennett DE, Brady AR, Herbert J *et al.* Drug resistant TB in England and Wales 1993–1995. *Thorax* 1996; 51(Suppl 3):S32.

13. Bloom B, Cole S, Duncan K *et al.* Tuberculosis: old lessons unlearnt? *Lancet* 1997; 350:149.

14. O'Brien RJ. Clinical studies of new rifamycins for the treatment and prevention of tuberculosis. *Int J Tuberc Lung Dis* 1997;1:S11.

15. Corlan E, Marcia C, Macavei C *et al.* Immunotherapy with *Mycobacterium vaccae* in the treatment of tuberculosis in Romania. *Respir Med* 1997;91:13–19.

16. Corlan E, Marcia C, Macavei C, Stanford JL, Stanford CA. Immunotherapy with *Mycobacterium vaccae* in the treatment of tuberculosis in Romania. 2. Chronic or relapsed disease. *Respir Med* 1997;91:21–9.

17. Durman P. Stanford Rook's 'miracle cure' for TB fails. The Times (London) 1997, 1 October 1997.

18. Condos R, Rom WN, Schluger NW. Treatment of multidrug resistance pulmonary TB with interferon-gamma via aerosol. *Lancet* 1997;349:1513–15.

19. Telenti A, Phillip W, Sreevatsan S *et al*. The *emb* operon: a gene cluster of *Mycobacterium tuberculosis* involved in resistance to ethambutol. *Nat Med* 1997;3:567–70.

20. Sreevatsan S, Stockbauer KE, Pan X *et al*. Ethambutol resistance in *Mycobacterium tuberculosis*: critical *emb* mutations. *Antimicrob Agents Chemother* 1997;41:1677–81.

21. Nash KA, Gaytan A, Inderlied CB. Detection of rifampicin resistance in *Mycobacterium tuberculosis* by use of a rapid, simple and specific RNA/RNA mismatch assay. *J Infect Dis* 1997;176:533–6.

22. Wilson SM, Al-Suwaidi Z, McNerney R, Porter J, Drobniewski F. Evaluation of a new rapid bacteriophage-based method for the drug susceptibility testing of *Mycobacterium tuberculosis*. *Nat Med* 1997;3:465–8.

Treatment of septic shock

S Sriskandan

Department of Infectious Diseases, Imperial College School of Medicine, Hammersmith Hospital, London, UK

Septic shock is the most frequent cause of death in USA intensive care units (ICUs) with a mortality rate of 40–70%, despite antibiotic therapy. Empirical adjuvant therapies directed either against infecting organisms or immunomodulation of host inflammatory response are sought-after. Recent multicentre trials of novel agents in sepsis, however, have taught us more about the pitfalls of conducting such large-scale studies than identifying new therapies. Sepsis and septic shock are aetiologically heterogeneous and it may be unrealistic to expect patients with post-operative Gram-negative septicaemia to respond to a given agent in the same way as a patient with streptococcal necrotizing fasciitis. Moreover, the magnitude of drug effect in sepsis trials may be small, and trial groups must, therefore, be sufficiently large for results to reach statistical significance.

There are a number of potential stages for therapeutic intervention in the sepsis cascade (Figure 1). Many such strategies, such as glucocorticoids and tumour necrosis factor (TNF), have already failed to show benefit in clinical trials.[1,2] Lynn and Cohen provide a full review of potential adjuvant treatments in septic shock;[3] the major clinical studies that are on-going or have been reported in the last year are summarized here.

Anti-endotoxin strategies

Currently, a variety of endotoxin antagonists are being evaluated, though their indications are necessarily limited to Gram-negative sepsis only. Bactericidal permeability increasing protein (BPI) is produced naturally by neutrophils and can both neutralize endotoxin and kill Gram-negative bacteria.[4] A recombinant fusion protein, rBPI, is currently being evaluated in the specific setting of childhood and adult meningococcal disease and preliminary studies are promising.[5] The development of other lipopolysaccharide (LPS) inhibitors, such as soluble CD14 and lipopolysaccharide binding protein (LBP), has been slow compared with rBPI.

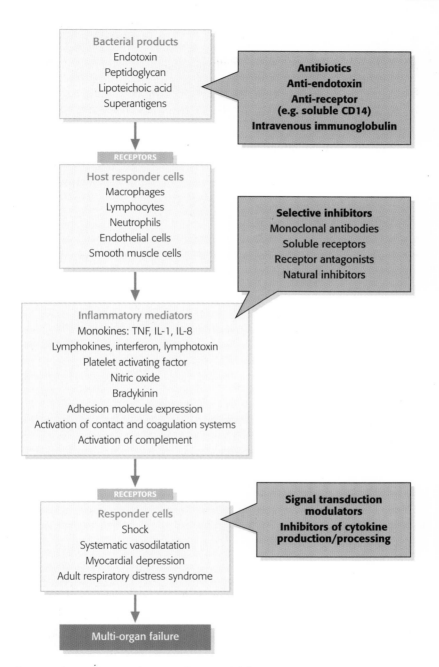

Figure 1 The sepsis cascade: stages for potential therapeutic intervention.

Naturally occurring lipid A analogues with reduced numbers of acyl side chains (e.g. LPS from *Rhodopseudomonas sphaeroides*) are known to act as endotoxin antagonists. A synthetic derivative, E5331, has been developed for use in clinical trials of Gram-negative shock and results are awaited.[6] Reconstituted high density lipoprotein (rHDL) is also being evaluated in this setting.

Anti-TNF-α monoclonal antibodies

Anti-TNF-α strategies have been of therapeutic benefit in a range of animal models of septic shock. The 1995 North American Sepsis Trial (NORASEPT) I and 1996 International Sepsis Trial (INTERSEPT) clinical studies showed that a neutralizing murine monoclonal antibody (mAb) to TNF-α led to a 14–17% reduction in 28-day mortality in patients with septic shock, but had little effect on patients with severe sepsis who were not in shock.[7,8] The suggestion that a pre-defined group of sepsis patients with shock may benefit more from anti-TNF-α mAb was, however, not borne out by a subsequent large multicentre study reported in brief recently.[9]

Soluble TNF receptors

Soluble TNF receptors (sTNFRs) circulate and can neutralize TNF during septic shock. A theoretical advantage of exploiting sTNFRs as therapies in sepsis is that neutralization of both TNF-α and TNF-β (lymphotoxin-α – a T cell pro-inflammatory cytokine) can be achieved. At least two distinct sTNFRs are recognized; sTNFR1 (p55) and sTNFR2 (p75). The p75 sTNFR has a lesser kinetic stability when bound to TNF compared with the p55 sTNFR. Experiments have shown that a p55, but not p75, sTNFR-IgG chimeric construct can protect mice from Gram-negative sepsis.[10] The difference in efficacy is due to persistence of biologically active TNF in the circulation of p75 sTNFR-IgG-treated mice, and is no doubt related to the lesser kinetic stability of the p75 sTNFR–TNF complex. Indeed, clinical trials of the p75 sTNFR-IgG in septic shock showed a dose-dependent increase in mortality in treated patients.[2] In contrast, a limited dose-finding study demonstrated that treatment with 0.083 mg/kg p55 sTNFR-IgG conferred a non-significant improvement in 28-day survival of patients with severe sepsis and early septic shock (though not those with refractory shock).[11] The results of a larger multicentre, double-blind, placebo-controlled

Highlights in **Treatment of septic shock** *1997*

WHAT'S OUT ?

- Monoclonal antibody (mAb) anti-tumour necrosis factor (TNF)-α
- p75 soluble TNF receptor (sTNFR)
- Anti-lipopolysaccharide (LPS) antibodies
- Platelet activating factor (PAF) receptor antagonists
- Glucocorticoids
- NSAIDs (e.g. ibuprofen)
- Bradykinin antagonist

WHAT'S AWAITED ?

- Recombinant bactericidal permeability increasing protein (rBPI)
- Antithrombin 3
- p55 sTNFR-IgG
- Nitric oxide synthase inhibitors (e.g. N-G-monomethyl-L-arginine)

WHAT'S IN DEVELOPMENT ?

- Novel antimicrobials
- Complement modulators (e.g. C4 binding protein)
- Coagulation modulators (e.g. tissue factor plasminogen inhibitor; TFPI)
- Nitric oxide scavengers
- Inhibitors of cytokine production/processing (e.g. metalloproteinase inhibitors)
- Signal transduction modulators (e.g. genistein)

study of p55 sTNFR-IgG in this subgroup of patients are currently awaited; preliminary results confirm that treatment confers a reduced incidence and duration of end-organ dysfunction, in addition to a 2.3-day reduction in ICU stay.[12]

Intravenous immunoglobulin

Toxic shock-like syndrome associated with severe invasive group A streptococcal infection is associated with a 30–60% mortality, even with antibiotic treatment and surgery. There are theoretical advantages to treating patients with both a conventional penicillin and a protein synthesis inhibitor, such as clindamycin, which inhibits bacterial toxin synthesis. There are no clinical data to confirm this, however. Intravenous immunoglobulin (IVIG) contains antibodies that neutralize bacterial superantigens, the purported agents of toxic shock.[13] There are no animal data to support the use of IVIG in streptococcal disease and no placebo-controlled clinical studies. Nonetheless, on the basis of clinical observations and limited case-controlled studies, IVIG has been recommended as an adjuvant to standard antibiotic therapy in this form of septic shock.[14] It seems likely that IVIG will also gain popularity in the treatment of staphylococcal toxic shock syndrome.

Nitric oxide inhibitors

It is hypothesized that excess production of nitric oxide (endothelium-derived relaxing factor) underlies much of the hypotension and cardiac failure seen in severe septic shock. Nitric oxide synthase inhibitors, in particular N-G-monomethyl-L-arginine (L-NMMA), have been successfully used in a number of animal models of Gram-negative shock.[15] However, the type of infection is a key factor; arginine analogues impede clearance of intracellular pathogens, and can have harmful consequences in rodent models of superantigen shock.[16] Nonetheless, a recent clinical trial of L-NMMA infused over 24 hours in septic shock showed a reduction in the time taken to reverse shock in L-NMMA-treated patients as compared with controls.[17] Mortality and morbidity end-points were not selected, and it is unclear whether L-NMMA is merely acting as an inotrope in this setting. A larger multicentre study with a longer L-NMMA infusion time and incorporating some 3000 patients is currently in progress.

The future

Antibiotic resistance is a spectre in any ICU; it is anticipated that molecular genetic study of pathogens associated with septic shock will identify novel gene targets for antibiotic therapy, that are expressed by pathogens only during sepsis.

Adjunctive therapy in sepsis (i.e. therapy in addition to antimicrobials) has been largely based on the assumption that endotoxin and TNF-α-mediated mechanisms underlie all cases of septic shock, ignoring the fact that 50% of cases of septic shock are related to Gram-positive bacterial infection. In order to understand and exploit the interactions between host and pathogen more fully, basic research is now needed to characterize the pathogenetic mechanisms that occur in more clinically relevant sepsis models. The complex interaction between host and pathogen may require a combination of treatment modalities, such as anti-LPS plus anti-cytokine. Combination therapy would target different stages of the sepsis cascade and, as such, may prove the best adjuvant treatment course to follow.

References

1. Bone RC, Fisher CJ, Clemmer TP et al. A controlled clinical trial of high-dose methylprednisolone in the treatment of severe sepsis and septic shock. N Engl J Med 1987;317:653–8.

2. Fisher CJ, Agosti JM, Opal SM et al. for the soluble TNF receptor sepsis study group. Treatment of septic shock with the tumor necrosis factor receptor Fc fusion protein. N Engl J Med 1996; 334:1697–1702.

3. Lynn WA, Cohen J. Adjunctive therapy for septic shock: a review of experimental approaches. Clin Infect Dis 1995;20:143–58.

4. Lynn WA, Golenbock DT. Lipopolysaccharide antagonists. Immunol Today 1992;13:271–6.

5. Giroir BP, Quint PA, Barton P et al. Preliminary evaluation of recombinant amino-terminal fragment of human bactericidal/permeability-increasing protein in children with severe meningococcal sepsis. Lancet 1997; 350:1439–43.

6. Bristol J, McGuigan L, Rossignol D et al. Anti-endotoxin properties of E5531, a novel synthetic derivative of lipid A. 32nd Interscience Conference on Antimicrobial Agents and Chemotherapy. Washington DC: American Society for Microbiology, 1992:337.

7. Abraham E, Wunderink R, Silverman H et al. Efficacy and safety of monoclonal antibody to human tumor necrosis factor α in patients with sepsis syndrome. JAMA 1995;273:934–41.

8. Cohen J, Carlet J. INTERSEPT: an international, multicenter, placebo-controlled trial of monoclonal antibody to human tumor necrosis factor-α in patients with sepsis. Crit Care Med 1996;24:1431–40.

9. Pennington JE. Issues in clinical trials of septic shock: industry perspective. 37th Interscience Conference on Antimicrobial Agents and Chemotherapy. Toronto, Canada: American Society for Microbiology, 1997;392:S59.

10. Evans TJ, Moyes D, Carpenter A et al. Protective effect of 55- but not 75-kD soluble tumor necrosis factor receptor-immunoglobulin G fusion proteins in an animal model of Gram-negative sepsis. J Exp Med 1994;180:2173–9.

11. Abraham E, Glauser MP, Butler T et al. for the Ro 45-2081 Study Group. p55 tumor necrosis factor receptor fusion protein in the treatment of patients with severe sepsis and septic shock. JAMA 1997;277:1531–8.

12. Pittet D, Harbarth S, Abraham E et al. Ro 45-2081 study group. p55 tumor necrosis factor receptor fusion protein reduces morbidity in patients with severe sepsis and early septic shock. 37th Interscience Conference on Antimicrobial Agents and Chemotherapy. Toronto, Canada: American Society for Microbiology, 1997;199:G35.

13. Norrby-Teglund A, Kaul R, Low DE et al. Plasma from patients with severe invasive group A streptococcal infections treated with normal polyspecific IgG inhibits streptococcal superantigen-induced T cell proliferation and cytokine production. J Immunol 1996;156:3057–64.

14. Norrby-Teglund A, Kaul R, Newton DW et al. The immunopathogenesis of severe invasive group A streptococcal infections: implications for therapy. 36th Interscience Conference on Antimicrobial Agents and Chemotherapy. New Orleans: American Society for Microbiology, 1996;318:S100.

15. Thiemermann C, Vane J. Inhibition of nitric oxide synthesis reduces the hypotension induced by bacterial lipopolysaccharides in the rat in vivo. Eur J Pharmacol 1990;182:591–5.

16. Florquin S, Amraoui Z, Dubois C, Decuyper J, Goldman M. The protective role of endogenously synthesized nitric oxide in staphylococcal enterotoxin B-induced shock in mice. J Exp Med 1994;180:1153–8.

17. Watson D, Beerahee M, Holzapfel L, Lodato R, Grover R, Andersson J. Multicentre, placebo-controlled, double-blind study of the nitric oxide synthase inhibitor 546C88 in patients with septic shock: effect on plasma nitrate profile. 37th Interscience Conference on Antimicrobial Agents and Chemotherapy. Toronto, Canada: American Society for Microbiology, 1997;200:G40.

Antiretroviral treatment in HIV-1 infected adults

B Ramratnam and MH Markowitz

Rockefeller University and Aaron Diamond AIDS Research Center, New York, USA

The treatment of HIV infection has changed dramatically. This is due to a better understanding of the biology of HIV infection, the availability of more precise methods to measure virus activity, and the discovery of potent, new drugs that target different phases of the viral life cycle.

The paradigm of HIV-1 infection and the goal of antiretroviral therapy

CD4-expressing cells, such as CD4-positive lymphocytes (T helper cells), are the main targets for HIV.[1] Upon viral entry, a cascade of events takes place resulting in the production and release of virions and the eventual death of these actively infected cells (Figure 1). The kinetics of infection are rapid; the half-life of free plasma virus is at most 6 hours and the life span of lymphocytes producing virus is slightly longer than 1 day.[2-4] More than a billion lymphocytes are infected and destroyed daily and their replenishment depends on the regenerative capacity of the immune system. The rapid replication rate of the virus, if left unchecked, ensures the emergence of resistance to antiretroviral agents when given as monotherapy or late in the course of infection. HIV replication clearly propels immune destruction and disease progression. The goal of antiretroviral therapy is to halt virus replication, thereby protecting all uninfected, susceptible cells from infection, and allowing all previously infected cells to decay.[5]

When should antiretroviral therapy be started?

The decision to initiate antiretroviral treatment should be based on the degree of viral replication, measured by the plasma HIV-RNA. A recent expert panel has recommended that all individuals with HIV-RNA levels greater than 5000–10,000 copies/ml should be started on antiretroviral treatment.[6] These guidelines derive in part from clinical studies that have demonstrated that plasma HIV-RNA is the strongest predictor of disease progression. When 1604 men infected with HIV-1 were followed over a 10-year period, this baseline parameter emerged as the best single predictor of

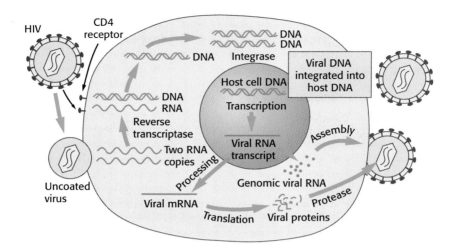

Figure 1 Replication cycle of HIV-1.

disease progression.[7] Importantly, treatment decisions should no longer be guided solely by the clinical stage of infection ('symptomatic' or 'AIDS') or the CD4 lymphocyte count (< 500 cells/mm^3).

Early treatment in primary HIV infection.

Primary infection is defined as the period surrounding HIV infection. It is associated with a burst in virus replication reflected by very high plasma HIV-RNA levels. Following this peak, circulating levels of virus fall to a level which remains more or less stable over time (i.e the viral set point). Compelling theoretical reasons exist for starting individuals on combination antiretroviral therapy as early as possible during primary infection. First, studies have clearly shown that the HIV-RNA level after seroconversion predicts clinical outcome.[8] Thus, treatment before, during or shortly after seroconversion may lower the initial viral set point and thereby improve the subsequent clinical course. Early treatment may also reduce the potential size of different infected compartments. Finally, as the virus population is most uniform early in infection, inherent drug resistance should be minimal.

Numerous studies evaluating the benefits of treatment during primary infection are in progress. Preliminary results suggest that combination therapy, using regimens including the reverse transcriptase inhibitors (RTIs)

Highlights in **Antiretroviral treatment in HIV-1 infected adults** 1997

WHAT'S IN ?

- Begin antiretroviral therapy as soon as possible after HIV infection
- Initiate therapy with a combination of agents including at least two nucleoside analogue inhibitors, and one or more protease inhibitors
- Use HIV-RNA to follow patients and to evaluate efficacy of treatment
- Continue treatment indefinitely

WHAT'S OUT ?

- Defer treatment until clinical deterioration or until CD4 count declines below 500 cells/mm^3
- Monotherapy with any agent
- Follow patients with CD4 counts

and one or two potent protease inhibitors, results in dramatic reductions in total body virus burden as demonstrated by studies of blood and lymphoid tissue.[9]

What antiretroviral agents should be used?

Currently available antiretroviral agents target two constitutive HIV enzymes, reverse transcriptase and protease. The various agents differ in potency, dosing and side-effect profile (Table 1). Eleven agents are commercially available and many different regimens have been examined in clinical trials. Current treatment approaches have derived from several recent investigations that have conclusively demonstrated the superiority of combination therapy to monotherapy.[10–12] In the Delta trial, in which 3207 HIV-1 infected individuals received either AZT alone or combinations of AZT and the other antiviral agents didanosine (ddI) or zalcitabine (ddC),

TABLE 1

Currently available antiretroviral agents: mechanism of action and adverse effects

Currently available agents in the USA	Adverse effects
Nucleoside reverse transcriptase inhibitors*	
• Didanosine (ddl)	Pancreatitis, peripheral neuropathy
• Lamivudine (3TC)	Diarrhoea, fatigue, headache
• Stavudine (d4T)	Peripheral neuropathy
• Zalcitabine (ddC)	Peripheral neuropathy
• Zidovudine (AZT)	Dose-dependent anaemia, neutropenia
Protease inhibitors†	
• Indinavir	Nephrolithiasis
• Nelfinavir	Diarrhoea, fatigue
• Ritonavir	Diarrhoea, nausea, asthenia, vomiting
• Saquinavir	Diarrhoea, abdominal pain
Non-nucleoside reverse transcriptase inhibitors‡	
• Delavirdine	Rash
• Nevirapine	Rash, transient sedation

* **Nucleoside reverse transcriptase inhibitors:** Phosphorylated by cellular enzymes and incorporated into viral DNA by reverse transcriptase. Once inserted into DNA, they terminate the chain by preventing addition of further nucleotides.

† **Protease inhibitors:** Inhibit processing of viral polyprotein precursors by viral protease enzyme thus preventing virion maturation. They are extensively metabolized by the P450 system in liver and small intestine and drug levels may be affected by other medications that either induce or inhibit the system.

‡ **Non-nucleoside reverse transcriptase inhibitors:** Non-competitive binding and inhibition of viral reverse transcriptase.

combination therapy produced 23–42% reduction in mortality risk and conferred a 23–36% reduction in risk of disease progression.[10] Given the dynamics of virus replication, monotherapy, regardless of which agent is used, leads to the rapid development of resistance (within weeks to months) and is doomed to fail. Just as two RTIs are superior to one, clinical trials in the last year have demonstrated that synergistic combinations of protease inhibitors and RTIs are superior to RTIs alone. For example, when combination therapy with the protease inhibitor indinavir and two nucleoside RTIs, AZT, 3TC or stavudine (d4T), was compared with the two nucleoside RTIs alone in a randomized, double-blind, placebo-controlled trial involving 1156 individuals, the addition of the protease inhibitor significantly slowed the progression of disease and decreased mortality during a median follow-up duration of 38 weeks.[12]

Viral suppression is best achieved by the use of a combination regimen employing a minimum of two nucleoside analogue RTIs and one or two protease inhibitors. If a protease inhibitor cannot be used, some advocate the use of a non-nucleoside RTI in the place of a protease inhibitor.[13] Patient tolerance, the existence of specific contraindications and drug cost will also influence the regimen chosen.

How should patients be followed?

The efficacy of a specific combination of antiretroviral therapy is best judged by measurement of the plasma HIV-RNA. Several technologies, including reverse transcriptase polymerase chain reaction (RT-PCR) and signal amplification, are available to measure HIV-RNA. It is prudent to use the same assay to follow patients over time. The optimum schedule of HIV-RNA testing will reflect clinical circumstances. After determination of one or two baseline measurements and initiation of antiretroviral therapy, plasma HIV-RNA may be rechecked at 3–4 month intervals.[14] In heavily pre-treated patients, more frequent HIV-RNA determinations may be necessary using an assay with a lower limit of detection of 200–500 RNA copies/ml of plasma. Plasma HIV-RNA will generally become undetectable within 3–4 months of the initiation of treatment in the majority of patients receiving combination therapy with three or more antiretroviral agents. A sustained three-fold increase in HIV-RNA levels despite compliance with therapy suggests treatment failure and may require a change in antiretroviral regimen.

The causes of antiretroviral treatment failure

Treatment regimens fail due to a variety of factors. The complexity of a given regimen (i.e. the number of pills, timing, and association with meals) and significant side-effects may lead to non-adherence, sub-optimal drug levels, and incomplete suppression of viral replication. In addition, despite best attempts at good medical management, agents added sequentially to failing regimens result in 'sequential monotherapy', which is an ideal setting for drug failure due to the rapid emergence of drug resistance. Finally, individuals with advanced disease (i.e. low CD4 cell counts and high HIV-RNA levels at baseline) harbour multiply drug-resistant virus populations pre-therapy, and may not respond to treatment. Thus, the importance of completely suppressing viral activity cannot be overstated. Clinicians should strive to design effective and tolerable regimens for individual patients, with careful attention to previous drug history and lifestyle factors that may interfere with the ability of an individual to maintain a regimen. Patients should be counselled on the dangers of missing doses, and the importance of maintaining dosing intervals and dosing conditions, such as administration with or without meals.

Can antiretroviral therapy eradicate HIV?

The current antiretroviral agents when used properly in combination appear to be able to suppress virus replication *in vivo* completely, and thus prevent the expansion of infected cellular reservoirs. However, latent replication-competent HIV still persists, albeit in low numbers. Several recent investigations using sensitive culture techniques have identified latent reservoirs of HIV in patients treated with combination therapy for 1–2 years.[15,16] Thus, it is clear that individuals will require continuing therapy pending new pharmacological and immunological interventions that can target and eradicate the last reservoirs of HIV in infected individuals.

References

1. Schnittman S, Psallidopoulos MC, Lane HC *et al*. The reservoir for HIV-1 in human peripheral blood is a T cell that maintains expressions of CD4. *Science* 1989;245:305–8.

2. Ho DD, Neumann AU, Perelson AS, Chen W, Leonard JM, Markowitz M. Rapid turnover of plasma virions and CD4 lymphocytes in HIV-1 infection. *Nature* 1995;373:123–6.

3. Perelson AS, Neumann AU, Markowitz M, Leonard JM, Ho DD. HIV-1 dynamics *in vivo*: virion clearance rate, infected cell life-span, and viral generation time. *Science* 1996;271: 1582–6.

4. Perelson AS, Essunger P, Cao Y *et al*. Decay characteristics of HIV-1 infected compartments during combination therapy. *Nature* 1997;387:188–91.

5. Markowitz M. HIV pathogenesis and viral dynamics. *Antiviral Therapy* 1997;2(Suppl 4):7–17.

6. Carpenter CCJ, Fischl MA, Hammer SM *et al*. Antiretroviral therapy for HIV infection in 1997. *J Am Med Assoc* 1997;277:1962–9.

7. Mellors JW, Munoz A, Giorgi JV *et al*. Plasma viral load and CD4 lymphocytes as prognostic markers of HIV-1 infection. *Ann Intern Med* 1997;126:946–54.

8. Mellors JW, Rinaldo CR, Gupta P, White RM, Todd JA, Kingsley LA. Prognosis in HIV-1 infection predicted by the quantity of virus in plasma. *Science* 1996;272:1167–70.

9. Markowitz M, Cao Y, Vesanen M *et al*. Intensive virologic assessment of aggressively treated subjects with recent and chronic HIV infection. International Workshop on HIV Drug Resistance, Treatment Strategies and Eradication. St Petersburg, Florida, USA, 25–28 June 1997. Abstract 126.

10. Delta Coordinating Committee. Delta: a randomized, double-blind, controlled trial comparing combinations of zidovudine plus didanosine or zalcitabine with zidovudine alone in HIV-1 infected individuals. *Lancet* 1996;348:283–91.

11. Hammer SM, Katzenstein DA, Hughes MD *et al*. A trial comparing nucleoside monotherapy with combination therapy in HIV-1 infected adults with CD4 cell counts from 200–500 per cubic millimeter. *N Engl J Med* 1996; 335:1081–90.

12. Hammer SM, Squires KE, Hughes MD *et al*. A controlled trial of two nucleoside analogues plus indinavir in persons with human immunodeficiency virus infection and CD4 cell counts of 200 per cubic millimeter or less. *N Engl J Med* 1997;337:725–33.

13. Conway B, Montaner JSG, Cooper D *et al*. and the INCAS Study Group. Randomized, double-blind one year study of the immunologic and virologic effects of nevirapine, didanosine and zidovudine combinations among antiretroviral naive, AIDS-free patients with CD4 20–600. *AIDS* 1996;10 (Suppl 2):S15.

14. Saag MS. Quantitation of HIV viral load: a tool for clinical practice. In: Sande MA, Volberding PA. *The Medical Management of AIDS*. Philadelphia: WB Saunders, 1997:57–74.

15. Finzi D, Hermankova M, Pierson T *et al*. Identification of a reservoir for HIV-1 in patients on highly active antiretroviral therapy. *Science* 1997;28:1295–1300.

16. Wong JK, Hezareh M, Gunthard HF *et al*. Recovery of replication competent HIV despite prolonged suppression of plasma viremia. *Science* 1997;278:1291–5.

Antifungal chemotherapy

TR Rogers
Department of Infectious Diseases, Imperial College School of Medicine, Hammersmith Hospital, London, UK

The formulary of antifungal drugs currently available for the treatment of systemic fungal infections is limited. Most of these drugs have been prescribed over a number of years and have well-established indications for their use. During the past year, several studies comparing the clinical efficacy of lipid formulations of amphotericin B with conventional amphotericin B have been reported. Interest has also been shown in the use of azole antifungal agents, particularly in the treatment of patients with neutropenia or HIV infection. A recent meta-analysis provoked considerable controversy over the use of these agents in both the prophylaxis and treatment of fungal infection in neutropenic patients; one of the major concerns with azole antifungal agents is the development of drug resistance, which has been investigated in laboratory studies. Several other studies have evaluated potentially valuable new antifungal drugs, notably voriconazole and the novel group of lipopeptide agents.

Antifungal therapy in neutropenic patients

Azole drugs. The use of an azole antifungal drug to prevent fungal infections in neutropenia is well established. Several large randomized trials have shown that fluconazole reduces the incidence of *Candida* mucosal infections and fungaemia in neutropenic patients; however, none of these studies has demonstrated any benefit against *Aspergillus* infection, an organism known to be resistant to fluconazole *in vitro*. In a randomized trial comparing the other available triazole, itraconazole, with fluconazole, no cases of aspergillosis were reported in the itraconazole group (n = 455) compared with five cases in the fluconazole group.[1] Although this difference was not statistically significant, it is consistent with the evidence that itraconazole is active against *Aspergillus in vivo*.

Amphotericin B. In patients who develop febrile neutropenia unresponsive to antibiotics, it is standard practice to administer empirical amphotericin B. The conventional formulation of this drug often causes nephrotoxicity, which significantly limits its use and compromises therapy. The new lipid formulations of amphotericin have, therefore, aroused considerable interest, since early studies suggested they are significantly less nephrotoxic, but as clinically effective, as the conventional formulation. In an open study of amphotericin B lipid complex, a 66% response rate was obtained in 64 adult patients with haematological malignancies treated with the lipid complex, 5 mg/kg/day, for presumed or proven fungal infection.[2] Nephrotoxicity necessitated discontinuation of the drug in only three patients.

In a randomized study comparing liposomal amphotericin B with the conventional drug in the treatment of febrile neutropenia in both children and adults (n = 338), a significantly better response was seen in those who received liposomal amphotericin, 3 mg/kg/day, compared with those receiving conventional amphotericin, 1 mg/kg ($p = 0.03$).[3] However, there was no difference between response with liposomal amphotericin, 3 mg/kg/day, and liposomal amphotericin, 1 mg/kg/day, nor was there any difference in response obtained with liposomal amphotericin, 1 mg/kg, and conventional drug. The incidence of nephrotoxicity was, however, significantly lower with both doses of liposomal amphotericin ($p < 0.01$). Current practice is to switch from conventional amphotericin if nephrotoxicity develops rather than use a lipid formulation as first choice, simply because of the greater cost involved. From the above study, it would appear that, for febrile neutropenia, a dose of 1 mg/kg/day of liposomal amphotericin is as effective as a dose of 3 mg/kg/day.

Prophylaxis versus empirical therapy. A meta-analysis of 24 randomized trials of antifungal agents given for both prophylaxis and as empirical therapy concluded that neither approach conferred any survival benefit in neutropenic patients, despite the fact that the incidence of invasive fungal infections was significantly reduced.[4] Clearly, the underlying disease and other complications of cancer chemotherapy have a significant bearing on the treatment outcome, so that any survival benefit from the use of antifungal drugs may be concealed. Only series with good autopsy data will reveal the true benefit achieved.

Highlights in **Antifungal chemotherapy** *1997*

WHAT'S IN ?

- Lipid formulations of amphotericin B
- Itraconazole solution for treatment of invasive aspergillosis
- Fluconazole for the treatment of *Candida albicans* fungaemia in critical care patients

WHAT'S OUT ?

- Fluconazole in non-albicans *Candida* infections where *in-vitro* susceptibility is unknown

Treatment of candidaemia in critically ill patients

Candidaemia is associated with a high mortality rate in critically ill non-neutropenic patients, many of whom are seen clinically in the intensive care unit. There is a consensus that all patients with documented candidaemia should receive systemic antifungal therapy. In patients who are haemodynamically stable and whose infection is likely to be caused by *Candida albicans*, fluconazole, 400 mg/day, is regarded as acceptable. However, in unstable patients or when the infecting organism is likely to be resistant to fluconazole (non-*C. albicans* spp.), amphotericin B is preferred either alone or in combination.[5] Routine antifungal prophylaxis is not recommended in this heterogeneous group of patients, as the incidence of candidaemia is still low and it is difficult to predict which patients will develop infection.

An important complication of candidaemia is endophthalmitis, which is commonly associated with the presence of a long-term indwelling vascular line. The optimal treatment is a combination of vitrectomy, intravitreal amphotericin B and systemic antifungal therapy.[6]

Antifungal drug resistance

In recent years, azole antifungal agents, and particularly fluconazole, have been used intensively in patients with HIV infection. This has led to the emergence of strains of C. *albicans* resistant *in vitro* to fluconazole, resulting in failure of therapy in oropharyngeal candidiasis.[7]

Some of these resistant infections can be treated with itraconazole,[8] which is believed to have good *in-vivo* activity against *Aspergillus*. However, there has been a recent report of three isolates from two patients with invasive aspergillosis, which were resistant to itraconazole both *in vitro* and *in vivo*.[9]

New antifungal drugs

A study of the new triazole, voriconazole, has shown *in-vitro* susceptibility in C. *albicans* isolates, though those with reduced susceptibility to fluconazole have correspondingly raised minimum inhibitory concentrations to voriconazole.[10] Voriconazole also has good activity against a wide range of mould fungi.[11] It is currently being evaluated in large clinical trials in immunocompromised patients.

The echinocandins and pneumocandins are a new family of lipopeptide antifungal agents with a novel mode of action, and activity against *Candida* and *Aspergillus*.[12] These drugs are also undergoing clinical evaluation.

References

1. Prentice AG, Morganstern GR, Prentice HG et al. Fluconazole vitraconazole prophylaxis in neutropenia following therapy for hematological malignancy. *Blood* 1997;90(Suppl 1):420a.

2. Mehta J, Kelsey S, Chu P et al. Amphotericin B lipid complex for the treatment of confirmed or presumed fungal infections in immunocompromised patients with hematologic malignancies. *Bone Marrow Transplant* 1997;20:39–43.

3. Prentice HG, Hann IM, Herbrecht R et al. A randomized comparison of liposomal versus conventional amphotericin B for the treatment of pyrexia of unknown origin in neutropenic patients. *Br J Haematol* 1997;98:711–8.

4. Gotzsche PC, Johansen HK. Meta-analysis of prophylactic or empirical antifungal treatment versus placebo or no treatment in patients with cancer complicated by neutropenia. *BMJ* 1997;314:1238–44.

5. Edwards JE, Bodey GP, Bowden RA *et al.* International conference for the development of a consensus on the management and prevention of severe candidal infections. *Clin Infect Dis* 1997;25:43–59.

6. Essman TF, Flynn HW Jr, Smiddy WE *et al.* Treatment outcomes in a 10-year study of endogenous fungal endophthalmitis. *Ophthalmic Surg Lasers* 1997;28:185–94.

7. Laguna F, Rodriguez-Tudela JL, Martinez-Suarez JV *et al.* Patterns of fluconazole susceptibility in isolates from human immunodeficiency virus infected patients with oropharyngeal candidiasis due to *Candida albicans*. *Clin Infect Dis* 1997;24:1214–30.

8. Cartledge JD, Midgley J, Gazzard BG. Itraconazole cyclodextrin solution: the role of in vitro susceptibility testing in predicting successful treatment of HIV-related fluconazole resistant and fluconazole susceptible oral candidosis. *AIDS* 1997;11:163–8.

9. Denning DW, Venkateswarlu K, Oakley KL *et al.* Itraconazole resistance in *Aspergillus fumigatus*. *Antimicrob Agents Chemother* 1997;41:1364–8.

10. Ruhnke M, Schmidt-Westhausen A, Trautmann M. *In vitro* activities of voriconazole (UK 109 496) against fluconazole-susceptible and resistant *Candida albicans* isolates from oral cavities of patients with human immunodeficiency virus infection. *Antimicrob Agents Chemother* 1997;41:575–7.

11. Radford SA, Johnson EM, Warnock DW. *In vitro* studies of activity of voriconazole (UK109 496) a new triazole antifungal agent against emerging and less common mould pathogens. *Antimicrob Agents Chemother* 1997;41:841–3.

12. Denning DW. Echinocandins and pneumocandins – a new antifungal class with a novel mode of action. *J Antimicrob Chemother* 1997;40:611–4.

Index

How to order

This *Fast Facts* book is one of a rapidly growing series of concise clinical handbooks.

Current *Fast Facts* titles:
- Benign Gynaecological Disease
- Benign Prostatic Hyperplasia
- Diabetes Mellitus
- Infection Highlights 1997
- Male Erectile Dysfunction
- Osteoporosis
- Prostate Cancer
- Prostate Specific Antigen
- Urology Highlights 1996
- Urology Highlights 1997
- Rheumatology Highlights 1997

For an up-to-date list of other titles in this series or an order form, simply phone or fax:

Phone: +44 (0)1235 523 233
Fax: +44 (0)1235 523 238